Getting Older Ain't for Sissies

A Conversation About Aging—
Its Challenges and Rewards

TERRI DIXON GAITSKILL

Copyright © 2025 Terri Dixon Gaitskill

Second Edition

Fulton Books, Inc.
Meadville, PA

Published by Fulton Books 2025

ISBN 978-1-63710-157-5 (paperback)
ISBN 978-1-63710-158-2 (digital)

Printed in the United States of America

To my children, Shari and Jackie, and my
marvelous "grands"—Heather, Jack, and Jenna.
I know that when I cannot "do" for myself,
they will be there to help. Love you all.

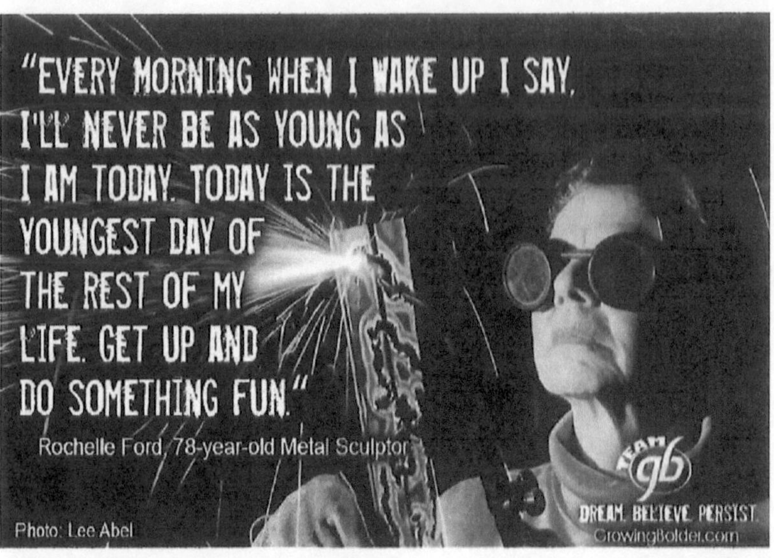
"EVERY MORNING WHEN I WAKE UP I SAY,
I'LL NEVER BE AS YOUNG AS
I AM TODAY. TODAY IS THE
YOUNGEST DAY OF
THE REST OF MY
LIFE. GET UP AND
DO SOMETHING FUN."
Rochelle Ford, 78-year-old Metal Sculptor
Photo: Lee Abel
TEAM gb
DREAM. BELIEVE. PERSIST.
GrowingBolder.com

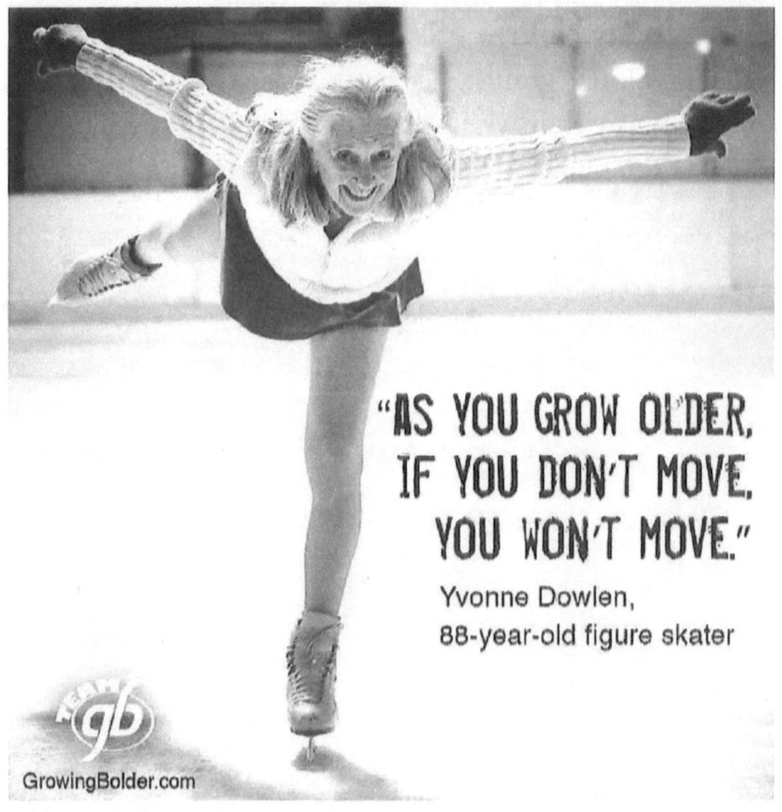
"AS YOU GROW OLDER,
IF YOU DON'T MOVE,
YOU WON'T MOVE."
Yvonne Dowlen,
88-year-old figure skater
TEAM gb
GrowingBolder.com

Nine Important Facts to Remember as We Grow Older

9. Death is the number one killer in the world.

8. Life is sexually transmitted.

7. Good health is merely the slowest possible way one can die.

6. Men have two motivations: hunger and hanky-panky, and they can't tell them apart. If you see a gleam in his eye, make him a sandwich.

5. Give a person a fish, and you feed him for a day. Teach a person how to use the internet, and they won't bother you for weeks, months, or maybe years.

4. Health nuts are going to feel stupid one day, lying in the hospital, dying of nothing.

3. All of us could take a lesson from the weather. It pays no attention to criticism.

2. In the sixties, people took LSD to make the world look weird. Now, the world is weird, and people take Prozac to make it normal.

1. Life is like a jar of jalapeño peppers—what you do today may be a burning issue tomorrow.

Contents

FOREWORD

I have been a nurse and a nurse educator for more than fifty years. I always wanted to be a nurse. At the same time, I also wanted to be a teacher. After completing my education at a hospital-based school of nursing, I got my license as a registered nurse. In the 1960s, there was a push for all RNs to have a baccalaureate degree. I, of course, did it the hard way. My program was called an "external degree" program through an accredited college. Coursework came through the mail—no online classes, actually, no computers. I completed the program while caring for a husband, two children, and working full time. I graduated with a degree in adult education (long story). This was very useful since a nurse is a teacher of patients, families, and peers. Next came national certifications in Neonatal and Maternal-Child Health. After working in obstetrics, gynecology, and surgery for thirty years and becoming a women's health specialist, I got a job teaching nursing, firstly to licensed practical nurses at a career and technical school, then registered nurse students at three local universities. I soon became a "generalist" as opposed to the "specialist" I had been. As a nurse educator friend of mine used to say, "We taught everything in the curriculum, from the womb to the tomb." It was during this time I got my master of science in nursing degree. My favorite subject to teach was

Gerontological Nursing, the care of the aging patient. I retired after more than fifty years. I woke one morning and said to myself, "Self, you are getting old, and you have a lot to share." I read an inspiring book by Dr. Atul Gawande, *Being Mortal.* I think it should be mandatory reading for all adults, especially health-care providers. He also has done TED Talks. From that realization, I started creating my "talks" relating to aging. These talks have been presented to groups at the local YMCA, churches, senior centers, and OLLI (the Osher Lifelong Learning Institute) through the University of Cincinnati. As I presented these talks, I learned from participants and varied resources about other topics of interest. What started as one talk has grown to nine. That thought led me to this book. I hope you enjoy what you will read. It is not intended to be a comprehensive medical book, but rather, a commonsense introduction to the changes we experience as we age.

Listen to the Aged

by Irene Burnside

Listen to the aged for they will tell you about living and dying.

Listen to the aged for they will enlighten you about problem-solving sexuality, grief, sensory deprivation, and survival.

Listen to the aged for they will teach you how to be courageous, loving, and generous.

They are a distinguished faculty without formal classrooms, tenure, sabbaticals. They teach not from books, but from long experience in living.

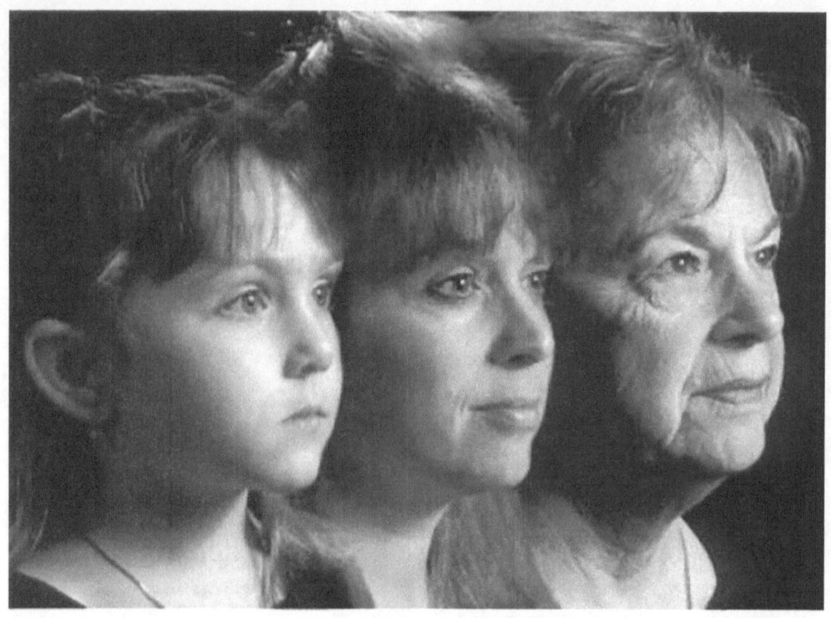

Factors Contributing to Long Life and Health

Definition of Old Age

- Young old: sixty to seventy-four years old
- Middle old: seventy-five to eighty-four years old
- Old-old: eighty-five to a hundred years old
- Centenarians: older than 100 years old

Diet, activity, play and laughter, faith, empowerment (not losing control of your life), and stress management are factors that directly affect how well we age.

CHAPTER 1

Physical Changes

Why You Sound Like a Bowl of Rice Cereal When You Get Out of Bed

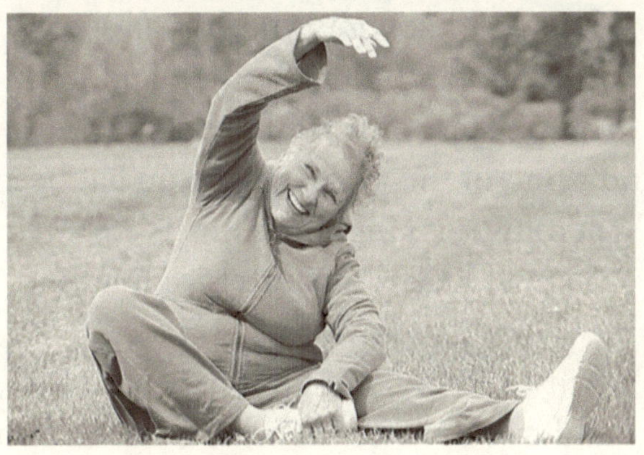

Physical changes during aging can impact nearly everything in life. Before you start this book, you might want to watch a YouTube video of Pete Seeger singing "My Get-Up-and-Go Has Got Up and Went" to put you in the mood. Feel free to sing along.

My Get-Up-and-Go Has Got Up and Went

Old age is golden, or so I've
heard said, but sometimes I
wonder, as I crawl into bed,
with my ears in a drawer, my teeth
in a cup, my eyes on the table until I
wake up.
As sleep dims my vision, I say to myself:
Is there anything else I should lay on the shelf?
But though nations are warring, and Congress is vexed,
We'll still stick around to see what happens next!
How do I know my youth is all spent?
My get-up-and-go has got up and went!
But in spite of it all, I'm able to grin
and think of the places my getup has been.
When I was young, my slippers were red.
I could kick up my heels right over
my head.
When I was older, my slippers were blue,
but still I could dance the whole night through.
Now I am older, my slippers are black.
I huff to the store and puff my way back.
But never you laugh; I don't mind at
all.
I'd rather be huffing than nothing at all!
How do I know my youth is all spent?
My get-up-and-go has got up and went!
But in spite of it all, I'm able to grin
And think of the places my getup has been!
I get up each morning and dust off my wits,

open the paper, and read
the obits.
If I'm not there, I know I'm not dead,
so I eat a good breakfast and go back to bed!
How do I know my youth is all spent?
My get-up-and-go has got up and went!
But in spite of it all, I'm able to grin
And think of the places my getup has been!

Did you sing? Smile? Laugh out loud? Good for you. You just exercised. Who says exercise has to be painful, strenuous, or boring?

I want to start with some of the normal changes that occur as we age. This is not a comprehensive list, but it will give you a foundation to understand why you feel and look different as you age.

Skin. Thinning, roughness, dryness, wrinkles, and lightening are expected. Loss of muscle tone and redistribution of fat is why, ladies, you no longer have an hourglass figure and why your upper arms, your "angel wings," continue to wave after you have stopped. Men, it is why you can still wear a size 34 belt when you have gained a few pounds. You are wearing it under your tummy. Thin skin can lead to bruising and skin tears, some causes are unknown, just waking in the morning can show new bruises. You might want to add a few pillows to keep from knocking the headboard in your sleep. If you take a blood thinner (anticoagulant) medication, notify your doctor if the bruises get bigger or do not go away in a few days. There is a need for less bathing—with mild soap, just the personal parts daily. A bath or shower three times a week (or if you feel the need more often). The inability to regulate the body's temperature is a safety challenge. You may be the only one in the room wearing a sweater. You might not notice you are getting overheated. This may lead to heat exhaustion or heat stroke, both of which are medical emergencies. Be aware of the temperature and humidity, drink plenty of fluids, and use a fan or air conditioner to maintain a normal body temperature. If your temperature goes up, you feel dizzy or disoriented, feel nauseous, drink fluids (not alcohol), lie down with your feet up, and loosen tight clothing and lose that sweater. If you don't feel better in a few minutes, call a friend or family member. Use your medical alert button or call 911 to get help.

Hair. Thinning, graying, and redistribution—ears and nose for men and facial hair for women. It happens. So men, have your barber stay on top of this or getting a grooming device. Ladies, there is nothing you can do to stop this from happening. Fortunately, there are several ways to manage it, from waxing, plucking, shaving, or laser treatments. The cause is the decrease of estrogen, the female hormone, that comes with menopause.

Discs thin. Loss of height. I have lost an inch so far. I bet you have had some loss.

Posture changes. If you had scoliosis (curvature of the spine), and it was untreated in your youth, it may become more pronounced. A hump on your back just below your skull is not uncommon but can be caused by a medical condition or medication. Have your doctor check it. The most common musculoskeletal condition of aging is kyphosis or the stoop shoulder, bent-over posture. It may result from a lifetime of slouching or a medical condition called osteoporosis, a reduction in bone density. Estrogen loss is the culprit here, also. Be aware of poor posture and sit up straight with your shoulders back and chest out (think a Marine at attention). Do this consciously while sitting, watching TV, eating, doing crafts, or driving. Your doctor may want you to have a bone density screening every few years as well as blood tests to monitor your blood calcium levels. Osteoporosis can lead to fragile bones that break more easily and take longer to repair themselves. Think posture, weight-bearing exercise, and a good, balanced diet.

Bones. Cycle of resorption (into the bloodstream) and renewal (into the bones) of minerals, especially calcium. Resorption is more rapid than renewal, leading to reduced bone density and increased bone fractures. Adequate vitamin D can help the body absorb calcium.

Joints, tendons, ligaments. Loss of cartilage means less movement and increased arthritis leads to pain, stiffness, and noise with movement. Cartilage in the nose and ears continues to grow, leading to facial changes later in life, especially in men. Ever wonder why the old relatives' pictures showed men with big ears and noses? Arthritis is common as we age—overuse of joints can cause this. I know it hurts to move those parts when it causes pain, but it also helps to diminish the amount of arthritis that forms. Anti-inflammatory medication taken twenty to thirty minutes before physical activity can reduce discomfort. If it can no longer be managed by over-the-counter medication, your doctor may recommend other medication or physical therapy. Just don't stop moving. Rheumatoid arthritis will require medical intervention. See your doctor if the pain and deformities of hands and feet occur or if you have a family history.

Muscles. Loss due to physical inactivity, changes in hormones, and reduced intake and use of protein. Protein is needed to make and repair muscles.

Circulatory (heart, blood, and blood vessels). Pause for a rudimentary anatomy lesson. The heart functions like a two-stroke engine run by an electrical circuit. Used blood enters the heart, shunts it to the lungs for an oxygen refill, then gets pumped out to the body full of oxygenated blood to nourish all the cells in the body. A problem with the structures of the heart or the electrical system can result in inefficient functioning and cell deprivation. Under normal circumstances, minimal changes occur if you have been taking good care of yourself. The heart can become less efficient with a reduced heart rate, stroke volume, ejection fraction, and oxygen uptake. The heart may not respond well to other conditions, for example, infection, anemia, surgery, diarrhea, circulatory overload (congestive heart failure). These may add additional stress on the heart, making it function less efficiently.

Valves. These are needed to make sure the blood goes in the right direction. Valves may leak and cause murmurs. Pre-existing murmurs may worsen. See a cardiologist if you notice chest pain, a fluttery feeling in your chest, skin around the mouth getting a blue tinge, or nail beds pale or blue-tinged. If you press on your nails, they should blanch white then turn pink within three to five seconds. If this is delayed, your doctor will want to know.

Respiratory. Loss of elasticity in lung structures, stiffening of chest wall muscles, and reduced ability to handle secretions (cough). Buildup of secretions may lead to pneumonia. Posture directly impacts your breathing effort. Exercise: Sit up straight. Take a deep breath. The chest should rise and fall easily. Now, slouch down and take a deep breath. It is more difficult to fill your lungs fully. You are probably not taking full breaths regularly, so your muscles between your ribs can weaken. Now, put your hands on your rib cage. Breathe normally. Now take a deep breath. Feel the difference? Help your body maintain as much efficiency as possible by doing this exercise frequently.

Kidneys. Responsible for excreting toxins, regulating water and salts, acid-base balance in the blood; very vascular, produce a hormone that stimulates bones to produce red blood cells and produce an enzyme to regulate blood pressure. Men may develop enlarged prostate glands. It is very important to have a doctor physically check regularly and have a prostate-specific antigen (PSA) blood test to monitor the health of the prostate. An enlarged prostate can cause delayed urination, dribbling, or failure to completely empty the bladder which can lead to bladder infections.

Bladder. As we age, the size of our bladder shrinks, leading to having to void more frequently. Many older people restrict fluid intake to decrease the number of times they get up to go to the bathroom, especially at night. This is a bad idea. It can lead to dehydration or an increase in infection. Women have a tendency to leak urine or lose bladder control when sneezing, coughing, laughing, or lifting heavy objects. This is due to weakened pelvic muscles. To strengthen these muscles, the ever-popular Kegel exercises are recommended. This involves tightening the pelvic muscles, holding it for a short time, then releasing the muscles. Do this while reading, eating, or driving. Make a habit of doing these exercises often. Sometimes, surgery can be very effective. If you have problems getting up in the middle of the night, you may want to explore the many varieties of incontinence pads on the market. If you take diuretics, take them in the morning so you won't get up frequently at night.

Endocrine system (hormones). Responsible for production and regulation of reproduction, growth and development, maintenance of homeostasis (balance), response to stress, nutrient balance, cell metabolism, and energy balance. One of the most common problem is for the thyroid activity to decrease as we age. Your doctor will monitor this with a physical examination and blood work. Abnormal levels can be controlled with medication or surgery.

Digestive system. Mouth and teeth—wear and tear can lead to ineffective chewing. Reduced saliva in the mouth can lead to dry mouth and bad breath. Digestion starts in the mouth as saliva contains digestive enzymes, so a proper amount of saliva is very important in this process. Taste buds decrease, and food does not taste as good as it used to. If you are on a salt-restricted diet, adding more salt is not recommended. Try using other spices—garlic, thyme, chili powder, onions, etc.

Teeth. Good dental hygiene is very important throughout our lives. It is even more important as we get older. Regular brushing and flossing can control mouth bacteria which could lead to periodontal disease. This can cause cavities, which can be painful and lead to dental care which can be very expensive as well as painful. Regular visits to the dentist can help keep your teeth healthy. Having to have teeth pulled or getting dentures can directly impact nutrition and can be very expensive. On the topic of dentures, your original dentures need to be worn consistently so your mouth can get adjusted to them. They need to be cleaned daily. It is not uncommon for gums to shrink as you age or lose weight. If dentures no longer fit, they need to be refitted.

Esophagus. Peristalsis slows, increased problems with swallowing, and increased heartburn. Let your doctor know about increased heartburn. This could indicate a medical condition that may need to be repaired. If your heartburn medicine gives direction regarding length of use and your heartburn doesn't improve, it is time to check with your doctor.

Stomach. Decreased movement of food and start of digestion (reduced stomach acid) and reduced volume. These changes can lead to a feeling of fullness even though a small amount of food has been eaten. This can lead to malnutrition. Maybe, instead of three full meals a day, more frequent and smaller meals may work better. A small healthy snack between meals can supplement the meals. A healthy snack is high in protein and complex carbohydrates. Try peanut butter or cheese on multigrain crackers or a piece of fruit. Sometimes, cooking for one or alone can decrease the desire for food. Recognize this and try new recipes from a cooking-for-one cookbook or invite friends or family to join you occasionally.

Small intestine. Absorption of nutrients occurs here and is reduced because of decreased peristalsis (movement of intestinal contents) or poor intake.

Large intestine. Eliminates waste, slows constipation as a result of medications, reduced activity, and reduced fluid intake. You may need help with constipation. Check with your doctor about which over-the-counter medications he recommends. Some increase peristalsis, some increase water absorption to help the stool move through the intestine, and some increase the bulk of the stool. If constipation lasts for more than three to five days and is causing abdominal discomfort, an enema may be recommended. An impaction (stool that gets stuck in the rectum) may occur. This requires a manual extraction, which is quite uncomfortable. Increased physical activity, increased dietary fiber, and increased fluid intake will help manage your intestinal health.

Nervous system. Reduced brain weight and size and reduced number of neurons. Subtle changes may occur in the very old. Thought processing may take a little longer and many experiences to sort through. Long term memory is usually not impacted. Remembering words and names sometimes take a while to recall. It can be frustrating but normal. Think how many "fun facts" you have gathered over the years. No wonder they take a while to sort through. Alzheimer's and other neurological disorders can make you worry. Statistically, the number of cases is declining, and there are medications to slow the progress. Keep your brain healthy with physical exercise, good nutrition, and brain stimulation (puzzles, word games, classes, etc.) Your doctor can test your mental acuity and order tests to identify changes in your brain.

Sensory changes

Smell. Sensitivity to odors decreases; implications for appetite and safety. If food does not smell good, you probably will not have an appetite for it. If your sense of smell decreases, you may not smell smoke or a gas leak and put yourself in danger. A working smoke alarm and carbon monoxide monitor are mandatory.

Taste. Decline in taste buds and saliva. Changes accelerated with dental problems, smoking, and medications. See previous information.

Touch: Sensitivity decreases. You may not notice pain as quickly and may injure yourself. If you are diabetic, check your feet daily for injury or wounds.

Sight: Presbyopia (age-related changes in vision), 95 percent of those over sixty-five use glasses for close vision. "Floaters," yellowing of the lens, cataracts, and fidelity of color reduced for blues, violets, greens. Bright colors such as reds, oranges, and yellows are more easily seen. Floaters are bits of debris in the field of vision. If they get too numerous or impair vision, see your doctor. Cataracts are a thickening of the lens of the eye. They can be treated. If not treated, it can lead to blindness. Glaucoma is an increased pressure buildup in the eye. It can be medically treated. Diabetic retinopathy is a decrease in vision due to blockage of the blood vessels in the eye. This can be managed with good blood sugar management: diet, exercise, and medications. Macular degeneration causes a decrease in vision in the center of the visual field and, if left untreated, can lead to blindness. It is a progressive disorder. It can interfere with reading, watching television, driving, and working on a computer. There are medications available to treat and/or slow the progress of the condition.

Ears. Presbycusis (age-related hearing loss). Hearing loss may be due to dirty ears (waxy buildup), sensory changes, or conductive (structural) changes. Your doctor and audiologist can determine which type you have and recommend treatment. Hearing aids may help with hearing loss. They are expensive and do take a while to adjust to them. Cochlear implants are increasingly used successfully when hearing loss cannot be treated with hearing aids.

Review—Presbyopia (age-related changes in vision), presbycusis (age-related hearing loss). Ever wonder about Presbyterians? The church is run by elders. (It's a joke. Giggle? Groan?)

Immune system. Decreased function and increased risk of infection. Signs of potential infection: sudden change in level of continence, sudden change in mental status, increased rate of breathing, increased sleepiness or agitation, and unusual paleness.

Reproductive health. Men—erectile dysfunction can be caused by medication, decreased blood flow to the penis, or some chronic conditions. Your doctor can speak to you about treatment options. Prostate enlargement has been discussed earlier in this chapter. Prostate cancer is usually a slow-growing and treatable form of cancer. The PSA blood test and physical examination can identify this condition. As men age, their sperm count will decrease as well as the quality of the sperm. A man will produce sperm until he dies and can still father a baby.

Hormones. Testosterone and progesterone levels can fluctuate. As a result, muscle mass and strength can reduce. The "mid-life crisis" can partially be attributed to these.

Women—menopause is the result of the normal reduction of estrogen, leading to perimenopause with the mood changes, irregular menstrual cycles, and hot flashes in women thirty-five to around fifty-five years old, and with it comes menopause (the end of menstruation and childbearing). This can be a good thing for women with endometriosis since the hormones for the production of the uterine lining stops, and the pain and discomfort of endometriosis ends. It can be a time of rejoicing because of the likelihood of pregnancy is over. It can also be a time of sadness. No more eggs mean no more pregnancies. Some women mourn this stage of life and may struggle with being "less than a whole woman." These women may need counseling to help them adjust.

Intimate relations. "Old people don't have sex" is a myth, and it is wrong. People still want and need some kind of sexual relationship and closeness until the end of life. As long as partners are healthy and in a loving relationship, this need remains; however, how it occurs may change. Based on physical limitations, positions may need to be modified. With arthritic changes, knees and shoulders may not cooperate for the standard "missionary position." Try different positions or methods that work for you. For lower hormones or "stuck in a rut" relationships come a reduced libido or sex drive. I love the words to Garth Brooks's song "Other Than the Night:" "She needs to know she's wanted. She needs to be held tight, somewhere other than the night." We are older. The kids are grown and need less of our time. We are retired or looking forward to retirement. Now is a good time to reconnect.

Medical conditions such as diabetes, heart disease, respiratory disease, and others may need medical guidance. Menopausal reductions of vaginal secretions due to hormone levels decreasing can cause painful intercourse. There are over-the-counter lubricants or your doctor can prescribe medication. All people need connection to others. The need for touching, hugging, and cuddling does not end just because we get old.

Medication Issues

Pharmacokinetics. Study of the movement and action of a drug in the body; determines the concentration of drugs in the body which in turn determines how well it works; the concentration of the drug at different times depends on how the drug is taken into the body; where the drug is dispersed; where the drug is broken down; how the drug gets out of the body. Think of the physical age-related changes and how that might affect the effectiveness of the medication. Comorbidity—having more than one medical problem at a time.

Polypharmacy. Use of multiple medications or use of multiple medications for the same problem. Twenty percent of the older population takes ten medications or more.

Risks

- Duplicate medications.
- Inappropriate medications
- After drug taken into the body: by mouth, injected into a muscle, or intravenously (IV)
- Potentially unsafe doses: Remember the reduction in the functioning or the digestive tract and the changes in other organs that may directly impact the absorption, metabolism, and excretion of medications. This can mean needing a lower dose or regular monitoring of blood levels of medication.
- Potentially preventable interactions.
- Multiple health-care providers (PCP, cardiologists, rheumatologist, pulmonologist, podiatrist, etc.) may not communicate effectively.

Your health is vitally important to you being able to age with a minimum of issues. Having a good health-care provider is important. Being an active participant in your own health is important. Have routine checkups with a doctor who you can talk to and will listen. Doctors have quotas and limited time to speak with patients during an appointment. You need to come to your appointment prepared. Bring a list of medications you take including over-the-counter and herbal remedies. Include the dose, route taken, frequency taken, and any problems regarding medication. Have a list of questions and/or medical problems you have had since the last visit. If you do not understand what the provider has said, ask him/her to repeat the information. Ask for information pamphlets. Take a family member or friend with you to help you understand what has been said or to remind you of a problem you have had should you forget to mention it. If you have vision or hearing problems, let the provider know. There has to be good communication, or you will not receive the care you need. If the relationship with your provider is not satisfactory, get a new one. I changed providers once—fired him. I was older, and he did not check my carotid arteries even though I have a family history of cardiac disease. I had to ask him to check them. He only checked my back for unusual "lumps and bumps" after I asked him to. I decided I needed another doctor—one that was attuned to the care of an older patient. There are doctors who specialize in the care of the older patient; they are called gerontologists. Their numbers are small but growing. You can call your local medical association for names of gerontologists in your area.

I hope you have enjoyed learning about the physical changes that happen to us as we age. These are general highlights, not all the details. These will provide you with basic information. Your health-care professional is your best resource for specific questions you may have. Do not be discouraged; it is not all doom and gloom. We can prevent or slow the changes with friendship, good nutrition, exercise, and staying involved.

A Youth Speaks

Until my grandmother became ill and needed our help, I really didn't know her well. Now, I can look at her in an entirely different light. She is frail but tough, fearful and courageous, demanding and delightful, bitter and humorous, and needy and needed. I'm beginning to think that old age is the culmination of all the aspects of living a long life.

—Jeannine, twenty-eight years old

A Middle-Aged Person Speaks

Nursing care of the aged brings one in touch with the most basic and profound questions of human existence: the meaning of life and death and sources of strength and survival skills, beginnings, endings, and reasons for being. It's a commitment to the discovery of self—and of the self I am becoming as I age.

An Elder Speaks

I'm ninety-five years old and have no family or friends that still survive. I wonder if anyone will be there for me when I leave the planet, which will be very soon, I am sure. Mothers deliver, but who will deliver me into the hands of God?

CHAPTER 2

Emotional Challenges

The year 2020 was an unusual time for everyone: the stresses of the virus, the isolation, the loss of friends and family, and the uncertainty. I have faith that things will eventually return to normal—a new normal but normal. The following discussion will address the universal emotional challenges we face as we age. Some of these challenges may be magnified at this time due to the virus. We need to recognize and address the additional stresses of the time.

According to psychologist Erik Erikkson, there are stages of life and developmental tasks we must successfully navigate in order to live our best, fulfilling lives. For the older person, those developmental tasks include:

- *Coping with change and loss.* Let us face it—the old gray mare, she isn't what she used to be. We have had experiences that have brought us joy and some that have brought us disappointments and sadness. Take a moment to reflect on these in your own life:
- *Establishing meaningful roles.* Did you ever notice that when you are in a social setting, you get introduced or introduce yourself by adding your pro-

fession or job title? "Hi, I'm Mary Smith, pediatric surgeon." "Nice to meet you. I'm George Carson, president and CEO of—company." "Hello, I am Jane Jones. I have been volunteering at the Aronoff Theater for the past ten years." Once you retire and are no longer in these roles, how do you then define yourself? What activities fill your day? My own mother-in-law worked for a doctor for many years. After she retired at age seventy-three, she said she "felt lost" and "didn't know who she was anymore."

- *Exercising independence and control.* Most of us will find our own independence and control over our lives changing as we age and experience physical and/or mental challenges. Do you have a plan in place regarding what those changes can lead to? Will you still be able to drive, live independently, and balance your checkbook? It is not always a pleasant thing to think about but being prepared can make coping with these changes a bit easier.

- *Finding purpose and meaning in life.* Do you feel that you have contributed enough? Do you now have time to pursue those interests you have been putting on the back burner? That sure beats sitting around and feeling sorry for yourself.

- Satisfaction with one's life and the life one has lived is gained by successfully achieving these tasks: unhappiness, bitterness, and fear of one's future can result from not adjusting to and accepting the realities of aging. Personally, I feel satisfied that in some small way I have contributed to the world through all the students I have taught and all the volunteer work I have done. Did I mention that I am a compulsive volunteer? I always told my nursing students that someday when I awoke from my coma and saw one of them, I would know I was in good hands.

Later-Life Transitions

These include retirement, grandparenthood, becoming a caregiver, or recipient of care. When these things come "too soon" or "too early," folks may have difficulty adapting. The speed and intensity of the change is the difference between a transitional crisis and a comfortable transition. Having a trusted friend (or friends) to use as a sounding board may be beneficial.

Retirement: About 33 percent of baby boomers have little or no assets. In some cases, the number may be higher based on economic downturns. Eighty-three percent of these Boomers plan to keep working after retirement. This could be due to boredom, financial need, or other reasons.

Sometimes a person so identifies with the job that when retirement comes, adjustment can be difficult.

Phases of Retirement

A person can anticipate thirty years or more of retirement. We could have 30 percent of our lives in retirement. We are living longer and healthier.

- Remote: future anticipation with little real planning.
- Near: preparation and fantasizing.
- Honeymoon: euphoria and testing of fantasies.
- Disenchantment: let down, boredom, and sometimes depression.
- Reorientation: developing realistic and satisfying lifestyle; downsizing the home when it becomes difficult to maneuver and maintain (i.e., the two-story home on two acres of land, stairs too difficult to climb, too difficult to mow the lawn, and maintain the gardens).
- Termination of retirement due to illness or returning to work: no more sleeping in, time spent in health-care settings, strain on finances, and strain on the caregiver.

Losses

Coping with losses: spouse, family members, friends, work, physical abilities, income, independence, residence, etc.

Death of a spouse is one of the greatest losses. Not only is the friend, partner, supporter gone, but many social activities are reduced due to feelings like the "fifth wheel" or you socialized because your spouse was good friends with the wife or husband.

Statistically, 66 percent of women are widowed and 86 percent of men. My husband used to tease me that men died sooner because their wives nagged them to death. A favorite phrase I like to share about this is: "Woman, you don't have to nag me. I told you I'd do it six months ago." One of the real reasons why women live longer than men is that they take better care of themselves, have regular check-ups, see the health-care provider when something seems abnormal, eat healthier, and get routine annual screenings in order to find and treat problems early and prevent complications. Getting a man to go to the doctor is like pulling teeth. I realize that these are generalizations, but in many cases, are the real reasons.

Widowers are more socially and emotionally vulnerable, leading to an increase in suicide rates. They remarry quicker due to loneliness and a need to be cared for. Ladies, we may have done our sons harm by not teaching them to shop, cook, clean, and do laundry. I know that sometimes it is just easier to do it yourself, but they need to learn these things, or they may be lost later.

Common Widower Reactions

- *Search for the lost mate.* I have a friend who lost his wife in the spring and ran into him at the department store shopping for his new wife's Christmas present.
- *Neglect of self.* Wife is not there to "nag" at him to eat, change clothes, bathe more regularly, or notice the button missing from his shirt.
- *Inability to share grief.* "Men don't cry." A bereavement group may be helpful. A protracted grief period may happen. We all grieve in different ways, but since men do not usually share emotions, it may be more difficult to "move on."

Loneliness

Loneliness is a universal human experience, and being the social animals we are, there are implications when those social connections are not satisfied. When the social connection is missing, the consequences are very real in terms of mental and physical health.

According to studies, the impact of people living in social isolation adds almost seven billion dollars a year to the cost of Medicare, mostly because of longer hospitalizations—a result that researchers hypothesize of not having community support (ARRP).

Loneliness is a killer; my brother was an example of this. He was in his fifties and morbidly obese, with a diagnosis of depression and anxiety disorder for which he was being treated. He had a heart attack (surprise) and quintuple bypass surgery. He did well, started eating better, and lost 150 pounds, then his anxiety and depression worsened. He withdrew from life, only leaving home to go to the library, grocery, and doctor's appointments. He became a hermit, not interacting with neighbors or family. He chose to sit in his recliner, sleep, or watch television. He lost strength and muscle mass in his arms and legs and began to fall. He could not get up by himself and called 911 each time he fell. After multiple hospitalizations for heart and lung problems, he was unable to live independently and went to a nursing home. Within two years, he died. He just gave up. His "hermitism" killed him.

Loneliness is a killer. It attacks our bodies and shortens our lives. It makes us more vulnerable to Alzheimer's disease, high blood pressure, suicide, and even the common cold.

Now the good news, becoming or staying engaged can add years to your life and decrease depression rates. Get involved in church, synagogue, or temple; join an exercise group at the Y or a fitness center; volunteer; join a book club, golf league, pickleball, or tennis group. Find someone or a group with similar interests like hiking, jogging, birding, or biking. Take a class, learn a new language, and play cards on a regular basis. It is important to find friends younger than you. The couples you have been playing bridge with for decades will start to pass away, and you will be looking for replacements. Travel, make and check off a bucket list, and make a "kick the bucket" list for your family to refer to after you pass. A close friend was very upset when she learned a cousin had died a couple of months previously. No one had thought to call her. I have contact lists on my phone, computer, and in an address book. Not everyone on those lists will need to be notified when I die. I created a list, my "kick the bucket" list of those I wanted to be notified and gave a copy to my daughters. They really appreciated having it.

In order to do some of the things listed, you need to maintain optimum health. Eat right, see your doctor regularly, take your medications as prescribed, whatever it takes. If you just sit there and watch the world go by, your body will deteriorate, you will get depressed and die sooner than later.

SO, GET UP AND GO FOR IT.

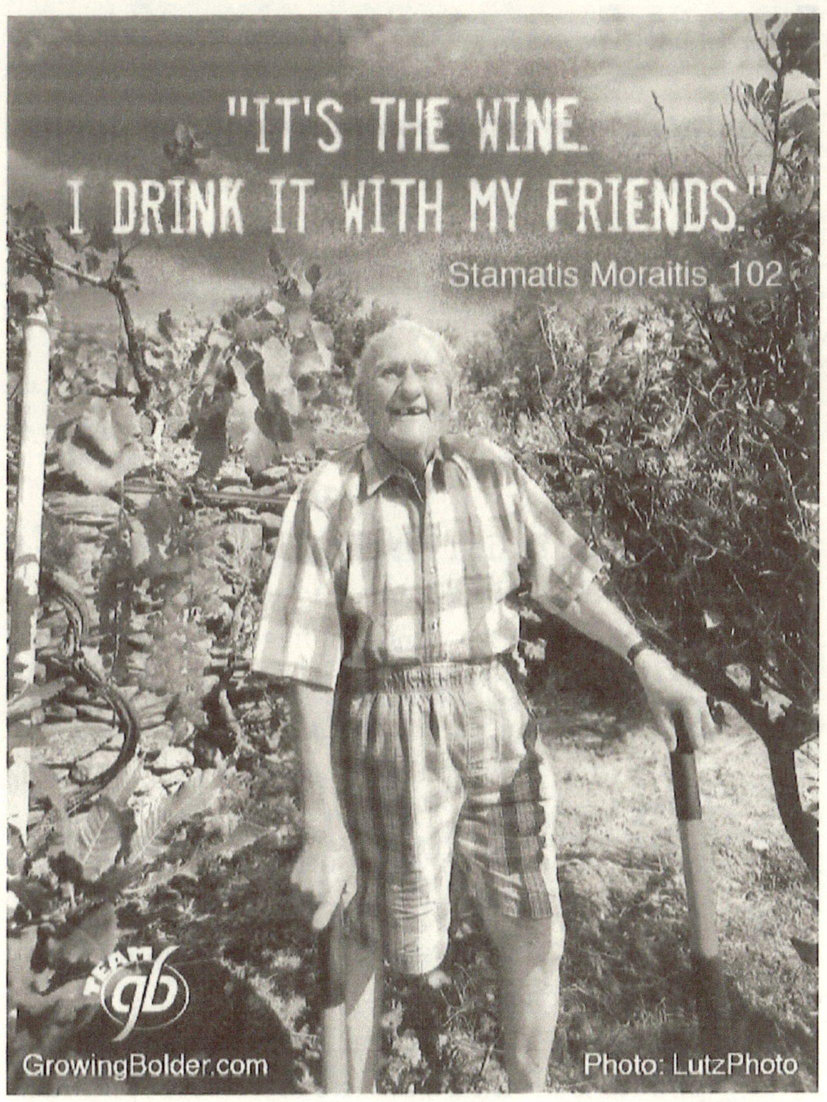

"IT'S THE WINE.
I DRINK IT WITH MY FRIENDS."
Stamatis Moraitis, 102
GrowingBolder.com
Photo: LutzPhoto

CHAPTER 3

Healthy Eating and Nutrition for Older Adults

As you age, your body and life changes, and so does what you need to stay healthy. Let's review some of the changes.

- Dental changes: normal wear and tear and ill-fitting dentures.
- Mouth: reduction of saliva due to dehydration or medications and decreased sense of taste.
- Slower peristalsis of the esophagus: swallowing difficulty and choking.
- Stomach: reduced size, reduction of stomach acid can lead to incomplete digestion, slower emptying of the stomach, and a feeling of fullness.
- Small intestine: slower absorption of nutrients.
- Large intestine: slower peristalsis; reduced hydration, fiber, and physical activity can lead to constipation and hemorrhoids.
- Changes in home life, health, medications, income, and sense of smell and taste may affect your interest in healthy eating and physical activity.
  - "The dishes I've always liked the most don't taste the same."

- ○ "Now that I live alone, it's too much trouble to cook for one."
  - ○ "I don't feel like going outside because I might slip and fall."
- Physical mobility: can you safely get to the store? Are you still driving? Do you have someone to drive you or shop for you?
- Finances: are you able to afford groceries, medications, and help? Are you living in a food desert? No groceries within easy access? Are you feeling depressed, lonely, or isolated? All of these can have a major impact on your nutritional health.

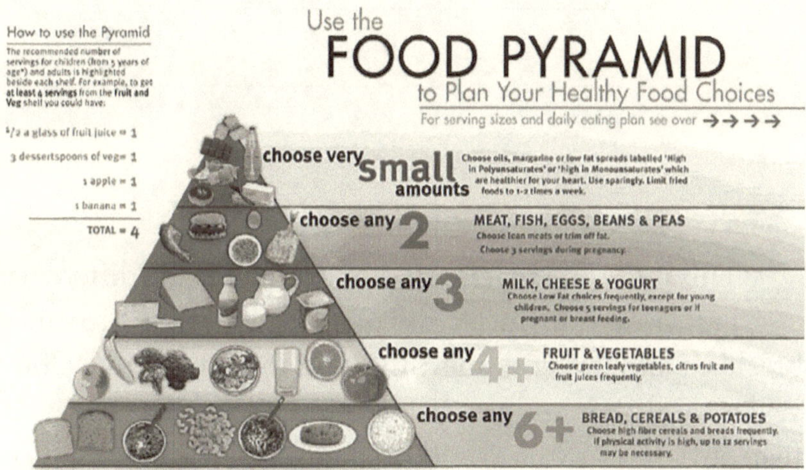

This is the food pyramid we all learned in school.

Modified Food Pyramid for 70+ Adults

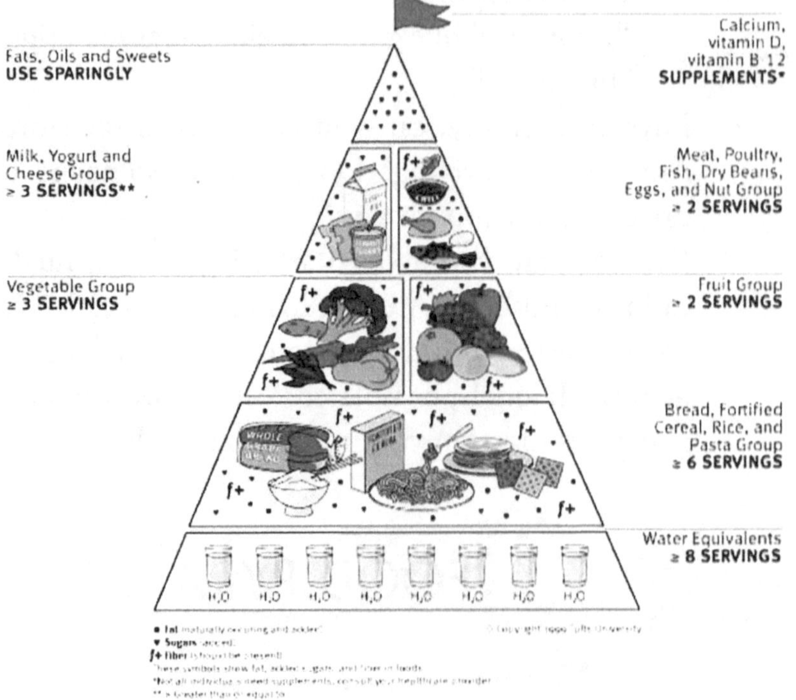

This is the one that is relevant now. Note the difference? Eat more lean meat, fish, and dairy, more protein at breakfast and less at dinnertime, and more brightly colored veggies and fruit and less beige-colored food. Eat more oily fish, olive oil, avocados, and less saturated fats; and eat more bran cereals and less refined foods.

A basic good diet for adults without other medical conditions is a two-thousand-calorie diet, nutrient-rich, and junk food—poor diet. Cardiac diets, diabetic diets, and other nutritional needs will be monitored by your health-care provider or dietician. The major components of a balanced diet are as follows:

- Fats: 20–35% of total calories.
- Carbohydrates: 45–65% of total calories.
- Proteins: 10–35% of total calories.
- Fiber: fourteen grams or a thousand calories.
- Calcium: for bone development.
- Vitamin B12: for cell and blood health. Deficiency can cause anemia. Causes of deficiency include long term use of proton pump inhibitors for indigestion, histamine receptor blockers (allergies), prolonged vegetarian diet, Metformin (diabetic medication), colchicine (anti-gout medication), antibiotics, anticonvulsants, and lack of the intrinsic factor in the stomach.
- Vitamin D: facilitates calcium absorption.

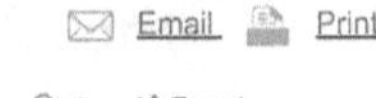

Reading Nutrition Labels

Sometimes nutrition labels can be confusing and leave you with more questions than answers. Have you ever wondered what a recommended daily percentage is? Or whether a product is really fat free or low in sodium?

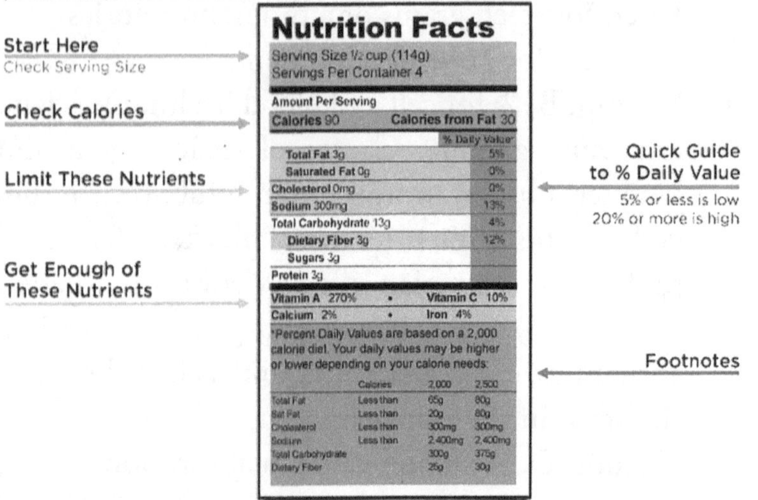

Companies are closely regulated when it comes to making statements about the food they sell. Check out our easy-to-follow breakdown of nutrition labels:

1. **Check the serving size.** This is what the entire label is based on. This tells you how much everything equals. It can range from five pieces or the whole package. This also explains how many servings are in the product. It's an easy gage to base the rest of the information.

2. **See the calories.** Now that you know what counts as serving, you can see how many calories a serving equals. If you are trying to cut back on fat, note of how many calories come from fat.

3. **Keep an eye out.** Try to limit the amount of total fat, cholesterol and sodium.

4. **Percentage per serving.** Strive to have low daily values of fat, cholesterol and sodium. Aim for higher daily values of dietary fiber and vitamins. 5% of daily value is low. 20% or more is high.

5. **Package claims.** Fat free means there are less than 0.5 grams of fat per serving. Low fat means, there are 3 grams of fat or less per serving. Low saturated fat is 1 gram of fat or less per serving.

First, check the serving size to see if it is the same as the one on the label. This is what the entire label is based on. It can range from five pieces to the whole package. This also explains how many are in a product. It is an easy gauge to base the rest of the information. Who knew that the Pop-Tarts serving size is one pastry? Why do they package it with 2 pastries? If you eat a double serving, you need to double the nutrients and calories. If you eat half a serving, you need to halve the nutrients and calories.

Calories. Now that you know what the total counts as a serving, you can see how many calories a serving equals. If you are trying to cut back on fat, note how many calories come from fat. Look here to see what a serving adds to your daily total. A person's weight and activity level help determine the total number of calories needed per day.

Total carbohydrates. Carbohydrates are found in such foods as bread, potatoes, fruits, milk, vegetables (especially corn, peas, beans), and sweets. Carbohydrates are the main source of energy for body functions. Talk to your health-care provider or dietician about the amount of carbohydrates you should have in your meal plan.

Dietary fiber. It is important to consume foods containing fiber from a variety of sources. Fruits, vegetables, whole-grain foods, beans, and legumes are all good sources of fiber and can help lower levels of cholesterol and thus reduce the risk of heart disease. It also promotes good intestinal health. Remember I talked about constipation being one of the problems that many older folks have? Consumption of twenty to twenty-five grams per day is generally recommended.

Sugars. Labels will indicate the grams of sugar in foods—both natural and added. Because sugars are a type of carbohydrate, the most important number to look at is the amount of carbohydrates for the serving you are eating. Talk to your health-care provider or dietician about the use of sugar in your meal plan.

Vitamins and minerals. Make it your goal to get 100 percent of each every day. Let a combination of foods contribute to a winning score. A daily vitamin and mineral supplement may be recommended by your health provider based on your individual needs.

Total fat. Try to limit your calories from fat. Too much fat may contribute to heart disease and cancer. Choose foods with fewer than 30 percent of calories derived from fat.

Saturated fat and trans fat. Saturated fat and trans fat are the "bad fats." Both are key players in raising blood cholesterol and your risk for heart disease. Fewer than 7 percent of daily calories should be from saturated fat.

Cholesterol. normal lab results for cholesterol:

- cholesterol: <200 mg/dL
- triglycerides: <50 mg/dL
- HDL (healthy): ≥40 mg/dL
- LDL (lethal): <100 mg/dL
- total non-HDL cholesterol: ≤129 mg/dL

Challenge yourself to eat foods with less than two hundred milligrams of cholesterol per day. Too much cholesterol can lead to heart disease. Cholesterol is found in food of animal origin such as meat, fish, eggs, and whole milk products such as milk, cheese, and butter. Certain food products that contain plant sterols or stanols can help reduce blood cholesterol.

Sodium. Too much sodium (found in salt) adds up to high blood pressure for some people. Sodium intake should be 1,500 milligrams per day or even lower, depending on your health. Most people with heart disease are encouraged to restrict the amount of sodium in their diet.

Protein. While most adults get more protein than they need, older people can consume less because of dietary shortages, inability to chew and digest meat, and slow absorption. Older folks may need protein supplements. These are better tasting if you blend them with a few ice cubes to make a shake. Even though protein from animal sources such as meat, fish, milk, and cheese are of higher nutritional quality than plant-based protein, it is also higher in fat and cholesterol. Use skim or lower-fat milk, yogurt, and cheese. Try to get some protein from vegetables such as beans, grains, and cereals.

Daily values. These daily values apply to people who eat 2,000 to 2,500 calories per day. If you eat less, your daily values may be lower (American Heart Association, Understanding Food Nutrition Labels).

The bottom line here is a good, balanced diet will keep you healthy. This is something we all know, but maybe choose to ignore. If you have a weight management problem, you need to ingest fewer calories (or more if you are trying to gain weight). We all still need the right amount of nutrients, vitamins, and minerals.

A fun challenge is to track your totals for the whole day. Another is to make sure you count all the calories in a meal—a Manwich label says it only has thirty-five calories in the can, but how many more is in the ground meat you added to prepare it? I have a vicious sweet tooth. Oh my, the calories, sodium, and fat on those labels. I rarely indulge in a full-sized candy bar. I like the information on the fun-sized candies much better.

Life Span Tips for Older Adults

- Eat breakfast every day.
- Select high fiber foods like whole-grain breads, cereals, beans, vegetables, or fruit.
- Have three servings of vitamin D—fortified low-fat or fat-free milk, yogurt, or cheese every day to keep your bones strong as you age.
- Drink plenty of water or water-based fluids (juice, coffee, tea, etc.).
- Ask your health-care provider about ways you can safely increase your physical activity.
- Fit physical activity into your everyday life. Take short walks throughout your day.
- Stay connected with family, friends, and your community.

CHAPTER 4

Heart Attack and Stroke

Why include a chapter on heart attack and stroke in this book? The leading cause of death in America is heart attack. Stroke comes in at fifth. Let's begin with a quick review of the anatomy of the heart. Refer to the illustration and trace the blood flow.

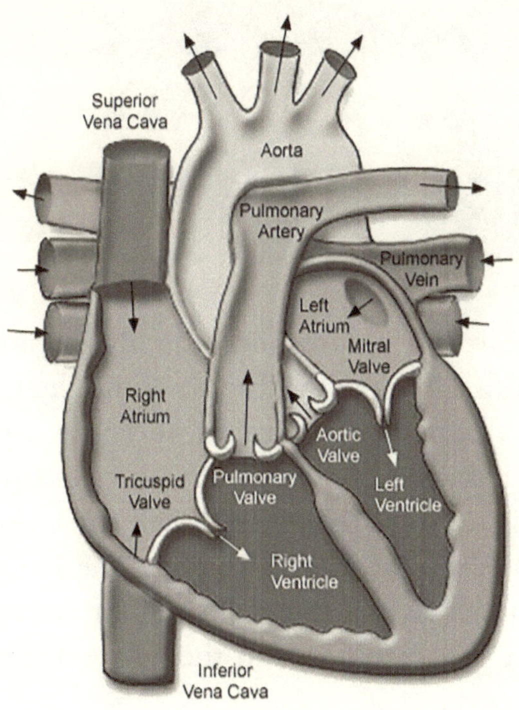

Anterior Heart Model

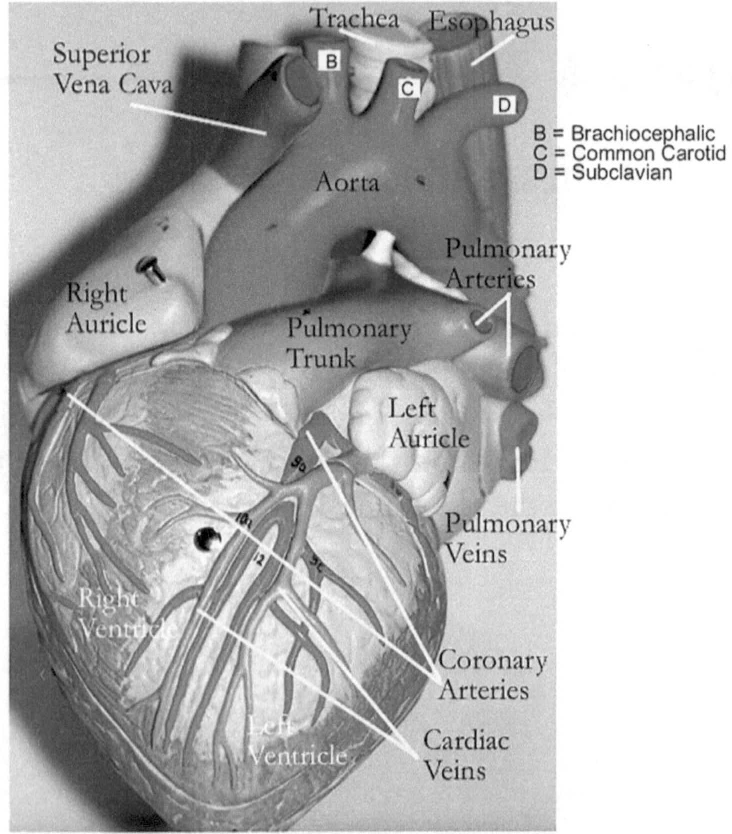

The heart is a hollow and muscular organ about the size of your fist. It lies in the middle of the chest, just a little to the left. The heart has four chambers: two upper chambers called atria and two lower chambers called ventricles. Their job is to pump blood. Between these chambers are valves to prevent backflow of blood. The heart has three layers: the inner layer is the endocardium, the muscle layer is called the myocardium, and the whole heart is covered by the pericardium.

How does blood flow through the heart? The right atrium receives deoxygenated blood (blood that has delivered oxygen to the cells of the body) through the superior (head and upper body) and inferior vena cava (lower body) and the coronary sinus (from the heart muscle). The blood then flows through the tricuspid valve into the right ventricle. With each contraction or heartbeat, the right ventricle pumps blood through the pulmonary valve into the pulmonary artery and into the lungs. Oxygenated blood (with oxygen) flows into the left atrium by way of the pulmonary vein. It then passes through the mitral valve and into the left ventricle. As the heart contracts (beats), blood is ejected through the aortic valve into the aorta and then into the systemic (whole body) circulation. The blood supply to the muscular layer of the heart moves through the two major coronary arteries. The left coronary artery arises from the aorta (oxygenated blood) and becomes the left anterior descending artery and the left circumflex artery. These arteries supply the left atrium and the left ventricle. The right coronary artery supplies the right atrium and right ventricle. When the left descending artery (which runs down the front of the heart) is blocked, it can cause a major heart attack—the Widow Maker. Interruption of circulation in any coronary artery can cause a heart attack.

A Quick Review of the Age-Related Circulatory Changes:

- Valve stenosis and elasticity (narrowing and loss of elasticity) prevents the valves from closing properly. Oxygenated blood and deoxygenated blood will mix, and the blood circulating may have reduced oxygen delivered to the body. Your healthcare provider may hear a heart murmur, and you may feel tired.

- Heart enlargement and decreased elasticity: when blood vessels in the body clog with fat (atherosclerosis) or plaque (arteriosclerosis), the heart has to pump harder to do its job. Like any muscle, if it works harder, it enlarges. The muscle wall will thicken, and the efficiency is decreased leading to poor circulation, blood clots, and increased risk for heart attacks.

Healthy Lifestyle

Reducing heart attack and stroke risk is all about attaining and maintaining a healthy lifestyle. The key lies in keeping your arteries (the carriers of oxygen-rich blood) healthy so plaque does not build up or clots form and block blood flow to your brain and heart.

Heart Attack

We have all seen the movie scene where the man gasps, clutches his chest, and falls to the ground with a heart attack. In reality, the heart attack victim may easily be a woman, and the scene may not be as dramatic. While men experience the pain in the left arm radiating to the neck or jaw, and the feeling of an elephant sitting on his chest, women may experience shortness of breath, pressure or pain in the lower chest or upper abdomen, dizziness or lightheadedness, fainting, or low back pressure or extreme fatigue. Even though heart disease is the number one killer of women in the United States, women often chalk up the symptoms to less life-threatening conditions such as acid reflux, the flu, or normal aging.

A heart attack is caused by blockage of blood flow to the heart. Treatments may include lifestyle changes, cardiac rehabilitation, medications (including TPA which needs to be administered within three to six hours of the onset of symptoms) to destroy the clot causing the heart attack, stents, and bypass surgery. A moment of reflection: if placement of stent(s) is called a PTCA, pronounced "pizza," and a bypass is called a CABG, pronounced, "cabbage," does that mean the pioneers of these treatments were hungry? I digress.

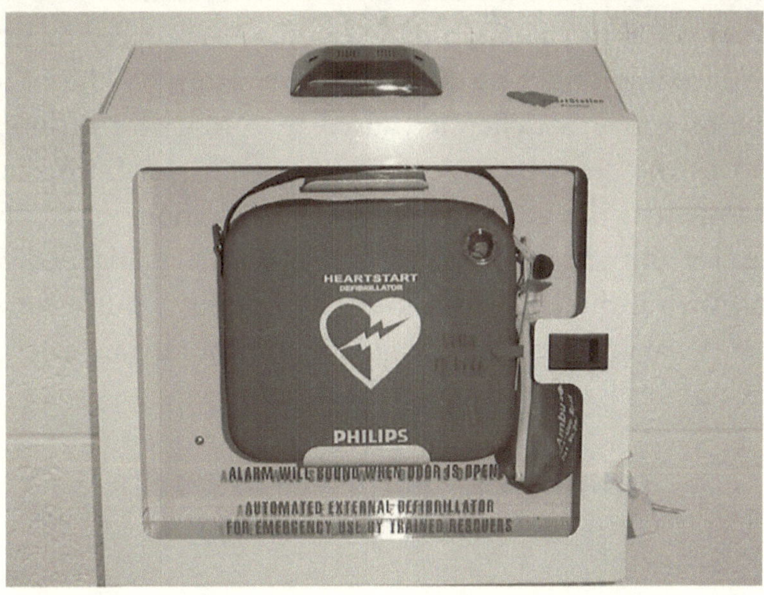

If you witness a person having an apparent heart attack, most businesses, schools, places of worship, and gyms have AEDs—automatic electronic defibrillators. I look around the places I frequent to be aware of the location of the devices. They are easy to operate and will give you step-by-step guidance. At least you will know where to get one if someone asks you to get it so they can use it. Getting certified in CPR may help you feel prepared to act if needed. The American Heart Association, American Red Cross, and local fire departments offer these classes.

Stroke

Stroke is the third killer of women in the United States and fifth overall in the general population. There are two types of strokes: Hemorrhagic stroke caused by a burst blood vessel in the brain and may require surgery to stop the bleeding and help minimize the damage. The other type of stroke is ischemic caused by a blockage of blood flow to the brain by a clot or piece of plaque. Immediate treatment is the administration of medication to dissolve the clot and restore blood flow. If you receive this medication within three to six hours of symptoms, your chances of survival and recovery are greatly improved. The clock is ticking—call 911 and get to the hospital!

Identifying Symptoms of Stroke
FAST

- *F (face).* If you are experiencing spasms, drooping, weird tics, or anything similar, look in the mirror.

Is one side of your face droopier than the other? Is your face off-kilter? Does one side of your face droop or is it numb? Ask the person or yourself to smile. Is the smile uneven?

- *A (arm weakness).* Is one arm weak or numb? Ask the person to raise both arms. Does one arm drift downward? Do you feel weak, tingly, or numb only on one side?

- *S (speech).* Is speech slurred? Is the person unable to speak or is hard to understand? Ask the person to repeat a simple sentence like "the sky is blue."

- *T (time).* If someone shows any of these symptoms, even if the symptoms go away, call 911 and get to the hospital immediately. Check the time the symptoms started. Do not drive yourself to the hospital. Time is of the essence.

You can get a refrigerator magnet from the American Heart Association to keep as a reference at home.

TIA

A TIA (transient ischemic attack) is a ministroke. When blood flow is partially blocked, often by a small blood clot, mild symptoms of a stroke may appear. After a short while, the blood flow resumes, and the symptoms go away. With a stroke, the blood flow stays blocked, and the brain can have permanent damage. TIA symptoms need to be reported to the doctor for follow-up.

Heart disease and stroke are very serious conditions. They result from poor circulation as the arteries in the heart and brain become clogged with plaque or fatty deposits. They can be reduced by managing risk factors. The main controllable risk factors are being overweight, smoking, and having high blood pressure. Other risk factors include age, diabetes, and genetics. We cannot control aging or genetics, but we can watch our numbers. Weight can be controlled by watching our diet and exercising. Your healthcare provider and dietician can help with that. Maintaining good glucose levels by watching diet and taking medication as prescribed can control diabetes. The bottom line is, keep blood sugar levels between 90 and 100. Keep cholesterol (less than 200), LDL (under 100), HDL (40-60 or higher), and triglycerides (less than 150) under control. Get stress under control—or at least managed. Quit smoking. Exercise regularly. If you have a family history of heart disease or have had a heart attack or stroke, make sure your doctor knows and watches your heart health closely. Keep your heart healthy, and it will keep working as it should.

The adult version of "Head, Shoulders, Knees, and Toes" is "wallet, glasses, keys, and phone." I'm at that age where my mind still thinks I'm twenty-nine, my humor suggests I'm twelve, and my body mostly keeps asking if I'm sure I'm not dead yet.

CHAPTER 5

Ageism

Ageism is the discrimination and stereotyping on the basis of a person's age. The relegation of older people to second-class citizenry. Stereotyping lies at the heart of ageism—the assumption that all members of a group are the same. Ageism is not a household word, or a sexy one, but neither was sexism until the women's movement turned it into a howl for women's rights.

Like all discrimination (including racism, sexism, ableism, and homophobia), it legitimizes and sustains inequalities between groups, creating layers of oppression in the lives of individuals and groups. This oppression is reflected in and reinforced by society through the economic, legal, medical, commercial, and other systems that each of us navigates in daily life. Unless we challenge it, we reproduce it.

Denial creates an artificial, destructive, and unsustainable divide between who we are and who we become. All aging is "successful"—not just the sporty version—otherwise, you are dead.

Like racism and sexism, ageism is not about how we look. It is about what people in power want our appearance to mean. Ageism occurs when the dominant group uses it to oppress or exploit, silence, or ignore people who are much younger or significantly older. It swings both ways.

"Aging in place" or "aging at home" usually means not moving to a nursing home or in with family. There is today a trend to want to stay in your own home. There are agencies and services available to help you do just that. A house can be fitted to meet the needs of people who may use walkers or wheelchairs, for example, new door hinges to maximize the width of doorways. We have all seen advertisements about "refitting" the bathroom with a walk-in shower or tub. Health-care providers can assist with medication administration, bathing, meal preparation, and other services. Stop by your grocery store or pharmacy and take a look at all the devices that are available. These things can be very helpful, and their numbers keep growing.

We are exposed to American culture's dumb and destructive obsession with youth. How do movies and other media portray older people? Hollywood is beginning to recognize the value of older actors. If we were to believe the advertisers, we can all look forward to erectile dysfunction and leaky bladders. Did you ever wonder why there are so many ads for medications in magazines and on television? It seems like two-thirds of the pages are for medicine you can't even buy over the counter. You need a prescription from your doctor to get them. Pharmaceutical companies spend more money on advertising than on research and development. It comes as no surprise that the cost of medicine has skyrocketed. If I see one more ad for Viagra or a skin rejuvenation cream, I will feel like screaming.

Science has leapfrogged culture, and society has not had time to catch up. Humans are notoriously slow to reframe perception and behavior. For example, education is for the young, employment is for the middle-aged, and leisure is for the old is clearly obsolete. We have yet to revise these structures in substantial ways or invent new ones. Current thoughts about aging include:

- "Wrinkles are ugly." I disagree. I earned every one of them.
- "Old people are incompetent." Ever heard of Justice Ginsberg?
- "It is sad to get old." Young people have student loan debt, joblessness, and unaffordable housing. Do not see them dancing in the streets.
- "Global wrinkling" and "gray tsunami." A terrifying vision of people looming on the horizon, poised to drain the public coffers, swamp the health-care system, and suck the wealth from future generations. Older people are a drag on the economy because of the way the economy is structured, and the structure has yet to be revised in order to take advantage of the vast, new, and untapped resources we represent.

The language is cold-blooded, and the trajectory is clear. Business reporter Ted Fishman states, "The high cost of keeping our aging generation healthy and out of poverty has caused the United States and other rich democracies to lose their economic and political footing." According to this train of thought, Western imperialism is in decline *not* because of the accumulation of "toxic" debt that threatened the global banking system or the effects of climate change or the stagnation of wages or crumbling public infrastructure or a workforce being left behind by the information economy or because the middle class is under siege, and wealth is being concentrated in ever fewer hands. The problem is old people. This is totally untrue, yet economists, politicians, and other policy makers are still basing their decisions for older people on these outdated theories. British economist, Phil Millan, exposes the reactionary analyses of people like Fishman. He states that the world's preoccupation with aging has nothing to do with demography. It has been used to justify the role government has in the economy and curbing the welfare state.

How does ageism impact health care? Ageism means less treatment or often no treatment at all. Because health-care providers deal with people at the more debilitated end of the spectrum, they are more susceptible than the general public to ageist attitudes and more likely to assume that aging and disease go hand in hand. The effect? Medical problems in older patients are frequently misdiagnosed or undetected. Even when disorders are correctly diagnosed, treatment biases or lack of information can lead to a lower standard of care than for younger patients (*This Chair Rocks*, 98–99).

- Physicians and nurses consider symptoms such as balance problems, incontinence, constipation, and memory loss to be inevitable consequences of advanced age instead of seeing them as treatable conditions.

- They are often dismissive of older patients' aches and pains. "At your age, what can you expect?" Geriatric pain is often not treated adequately.

- Findings suggest that physicians communicate better with younger patients and give older patients less time.

- Physicians often fail to account for age-related changes in the way older bodies absorb and eliminate medication, to check for side effects, and to consider the effects of being on multiple medications (Pretorius, Gataric, et al. 2013). Many older adults, especially nursing home residents, are dangerously overmedicated.

- This bias is reflected in public policy. The National Institutes of Health (NIH) Revitalization Act of 1993 mandated the inclusion of women and minorities in federally funded clinical trials, but not a lot of people over sixty-five, although they take many more medications. People over eighty-five make up the fastest-growing segment of the population, yet the prototypical patient in drug trials is a young person.

- Many doctors assume that older patients are not sexually active and do not ask about sexual histories or routinely screen for sexually transmitted diseases.

- Secondary preventive screening programs such as cancer screenings are often overlooked in older adults and may fail to offer adequate preventative counseling to their older patients.

Ageism in the Workplace

It is time to end the last acceptable bias. People report being "targeted in my fifties, then kicked out," "treated like I was senile," "passed over because I was nearing retirement," and "berated and being called a waste of time" (AARP 2020).

Age discrimination cases are difficult to prove. Job postings may include things like "recent college graduate" in order to attract younger applicants. These are illegal.

It is embarrassing to be called older until we stop being embarrassed about it, and it is not healthy to go through life dreading the future. The longer we live, the more different we are from one another. Think about it. Yet we think of everyone in a retirement home as the same age—old—when they can span four decades. Can you imagine thinking that way about twenty- to sixty-year-olds? Have you ever rejected a haircut, relationship, or outing because it was not age-appropriate? For adults, there is no such thing. These behaviors are ageist. We all do it, and we cannot change bias unless we are aware of it. Nobody is born "ageist," but it starts in early childhood, around the time attitudes toward race and gender start to form because negative messages about late life bombard us from the media and popular culture at every turn.

According to Ashton Applewhite, author of *This Chair Rocks*, older people can be the most ageist of all because we have had a lifetime to internalize these messages and never thought to change them. Acknowledge and stop colluding—senior moment quips, for example. I stopped making them when I realized that when I lost the car keys in high school, I didn't call it a "junior moment." I stopped blaming my aching knee on being in my seventies. My other knee is just as old, but it doesn't hurt.

Why add another "ism" to the list when there are so many, racism in particular, call for action? Here is the thing: we don't have to choose. When we make the world a better place to grow old, we make it a better place to be from somewhere else, to be a person with a disability, to be nonrich, to be queer, and to be nonwhite. And when we show up at all ages for whatever cause matters to us—save the whales, save the democracy—we not only make that effort more effective, but we dismantle ageism in the process.

If this information has piqued your interest, you can learn more about it by reading Ashton Applewhite's book *This Chair Rocks: A Manifest Against Ageism* or go to her website, TED talks, and other information on Google.

Chapter 6

Caring for the Caregiver

Caring can be a short-term or a long-term responsibility. For both, there may be a need to make many adjustments—work, family, medical equipment or procedures, and more. The way to make this easier on the caregiver is to be informed and to be educated about the needs of the person to be cared for. Ask questions, practice tasks with supervision until you feel comfortable, and use resources.

Caregiving for long-term needs requires planning, communication, and support. Caregiving is associated with increased levels of depression and anxiety, poorer self-reported physical health, compromised immune system, and increased mortality and stress reaction.

Suggestions for caregivers:

- Educate yourself about the disease or medical condition.
- Find health-care professionals who understand the disease/condition.
- Consult with other experts in order to plan for future needs—financial and legal.
- Tap social and family resources for assistance.
- Find a confidant or get professional counseling.

- Take time for exercising or relaxing.
- Use community resource—senior centers, senior day care, respite care.
- Maintain your sense of humor.
- Explore religious beliefs and spiritual values.
- Set realistic goals.

I know caregiving can be exhausting and stressful. Please remember, you are not alone. Do not be afraid to ask for help. Your needs are as important as those of the person you are caring for.

Reported Caregiver Needs:

- Finding time for myself
- Keeping the person I care for safe
- Balancing work and family responsibilities
- Managing physical and emotional stress
- Finding easy and satisfying activities to use with the care recipient
- Learning how to talk with healthcare providers
- Making end-of-life decisions
- Moving or lifting, bathing, and dressing
- Negotiating health care, home, and community resources
- Managing complex medication schedules or high-tech equipment
- Choosing a home health agency, assisted living, or skilled nursing facility
- Managing incontinence or toileting problems
- Finding non-English educational material

This is quite a list. Where to start?

Make a Plan

- Start the conversation: sooner than later. Search "conversations of a lifetime" to help you get started. The conversation does not need to be complete with the first attempt. My oldest daughter understands and is on the same page as I am. My younger daughter is not ready to talk about these possibilities yet.
- Form your team.
- Make a plan.
- Find support.
- Care for yourself.
- Counter resistance.

Contact AARP for helpful resources. A helpful resource is AARP's *A Planning Guide for Families* at www.aaro.org/caregiving or call 877-333-5885.

Start the conversation. Many people wait until a crisis occurs before they talk about their values and preferences. If you wait to have this conversation, your decisions may be driven by assumptions.

Form your team. No one should try to deal with the responsibilities of caregiving alone. Other family members, friends, colleagues, clubs, and religious affiliations can be resources too.

Make a plan. Putting together a family caregiver plan now can help you respond more quickly and effectively. It can provide peace of mind.

Find support. Many issues arise during your caregiving experience that require additional information or resources.

Care for yourself. It is very easy to forget about your own needs. Keeping up your energy and maintaining your own health are critical in order to care for others. It is as important to make a plan of care for yourself as it is to make a plan of care for others.

CHAPTER 7

Elder Abuse

I noticed a friend seemed really upset. When I asked her what I was wrong, she began to tell me about her older friend, Sally, who was in a nursing home and miserable. Sally's family did not have time or did not want to help her with shopping or even visiting. Sally's family decided that she was unable to live alone and admitted her to a nursing home. A few weeks later, Sally was telling my friend about her daughter's new car and kitchen renovation. My friend drove by Sally's house and found that it had been sold. Her friend was unaware that her family had sold her house and was using the money for themselves.

Phil, a seventy-five-year-old retired teacher, forgets the boiling soup, and the kitchen catches fire.

Carol receives an eviction notice after giving rent money to her nephew.

Laura thinks her sixty-five-year-old mother's mental confusion is stubbornness. Laura continually threatens her mother with nursing home placement.

Michael slaps his eighty-year-old grandmother for urinating on the carpet

Sam loves his eighty-year-old wife, Sarah, but is too weak to lift her to change her soiled sheets (Hamilton County Job and Family Services).

These situations illustrate the complex and growing problem of elder abuse. The Committee on Aging estimates that one in twenty older adults is abused each year. As the American population continues to grow older, the number of elder abuse cases is expected to rise,

Elder mistreatment is a complex phenomenon that includes abuse, exploitation, and negligence. While the exact definition varies somewhat, it always means harm that is caused by someone in a caregiving or trust relationship. Mistreatment of older, frail, and vulnerable adults is found in all socioeconomic, racial, and ethnic groups in the US and around the globe. Elder mistreatment implies that the recipient of the mistreatment is in a situation or condition in which the ability to protect oneself is limited in some way. Otherwise, the actions are more accurately described as domestic violence, sexual assault, or fraud.

Types of Elder Mistreatment

Physical abuse. The use of physical force that may result in bodily injury, physical pain, or impairment, any nonaccidental conduct that causes bodily harm.

Sexual abuse. Nonconsensual sexual contact of any kind with an elderly person, including those persons unable to give consent.

Emotional or psychological abuse. The deliberate infliction of pain, anguish, or distress through verbal or nonverbal acts, including intimidation or enforced isolation.

Medical abuse. Subjecting a person to unwanted medical treatment or procedures; medical neglect occurs when a medically necessary and desired treatment is withheld.

Financial or material abuse or exploitation. The illegal or improper use of an elder's funds, property, or assets.

Neglect. The refusal or failure to fulfill any part of a person's previously agreed obligation or duties to an elder dependent on the person for care or assistance. The daily living needs are not met by the caregiver. It can be intentional or unintentional.

Abandonment. The desertion of an elder by an individual who had assumed responsibility of providing care or assistance.

Why Does Abuse Occur?

Most older adults eventually need help with tasks such as meals, housekeeping, shopping, etc. Family members provide the majority of that care. Only 5 percent of older adults are living in nursing homes. Caring for an elderly person can be overwhelming or become physically impossible. Most families care for elders with love and respect, but when abuse occurs, a family member or caregiver is usually involved.

Why Don't Older Adults Ask for Help?

Only one in six cases of elder abuse is reported. Abused elders rarely tell because of

- shame or embarrassment;
- fear of retaliation (think of the movie *Happy Gilmore* with Adam Sandler, his grandmother, and her caregiver);

- sense of resignation or powerlessness;
- family loyalty;
- lack of credibility; and
- fear of nursing home or institution.

The Ohio Department of Job and Family Services collected data for all eighty-eight counties in Ohio. All states collect similar data. The statistics show that for 2018 from July 1, 2017, to June 30, 2018, a total of 19,492 reports of abuse, neglect, or exploitation were reported for adults over the age of eighteen. Of the *19,492* reported, *14,597 were reports for adults age sixty or over.*

There are laws in the state revised code that cover interventions and third-party decision makers, such as guardianship, conservatorship, and Advance Directive. If elder abuse is suspected, a formal report can be made, anonymously if desired. Doctors, nurses, and other health-care providers are mandatory reporters, which means if abuse is suspected, a formal report must be made. Reports are made to the Adult Protective Services agency through Job and Family Services. States usually have a toll-free number for reporting.

As a caring friend, we can check on our elderly regularly. A phone call or visit is a treat for those who live alone. Having regular contact such as enjoying a ride or sharing a meal can give the elder a chance to share if there are "things that are not right." There are agencies and services available to help or relieve the burden of caregiving. If you are the victim of abuse, report it yourself. Your health and life may depend on it.

CHAPTER 8

Conversations for Advance Care Planning

Information given is informative in nature. It is not meant to be legal or financial advice. I am not a lawyer or a financial professional. The perspective is that of health-care providers.

Have you ever gotten a piece of "junk mail" that made you stop and think? I did, and it turned out to be the beginning of this conversation. I got a piece of paper from a local funeral home. It gave information about the cost of various end of life services and encouraged the recipient to contact them with questions. Of course, I had questions. I made the call, met some delightful and knowledgeable people, and created this talk. The first time I gave this talk, a representative from the funeral home came with me and answered a boatload of questions. A pastor friend of mine shared her file of "Advance Care Directives for Spiritual Care." I will share some of this information later. I have a friend, Rebecca Pace, CPA, who has shared a workbook she created called *A Parting Gift*. In it are places to address the practical information your family will need when you are no longer here. Things such as: who cared for your dog when you went on vacation, who has a key to your house, where to find all of your passwords, name and contact information to your financial advisor and lawyer, etc. You can find similar workbooks in those catalogs that come in the mail. Another thing to think about is to create a list of those people you would like to be notified when you pass. I have contacts on my phone and computer as well as an address book. Not everyone needs to be notified. I have created a "Kick the Bucket" List for my family for this purpose. I have a friend who was very upset to hear after a couple of months that her cousin had passed away. If the family had a "kick the bucket" list, she would have heard in a timelier manner.

As a teacher, I like to include some historical perspectives when starting a topic. In 1990, the Patient Self-Determination Act was passed by Congress in an attempt to improve the end-of-life experience in the United States. The intended purpose of this was to inform patients of their rights regarding decisions dictating the future—their future medical care. Prior to this, the doctor was in charge of the care plan, a kind of paternalistic approach.

From this legislation came concepts such as Advance Care Planning, Advanced Directives, and Durable Power of Attorney for Healthcare and the Living Will, not to be confused with the Last Will and Testament. Advance Directives are the documents that state what is to happen if you are unable to speak for yourself, for example, dementia or Alzheimer's, or debilitating stroke. Advance care planning is the process of thinking through thoughts and values about end-of-life care, having the important crucial conversations with others and putting them to paper in the document.

Topics in Advance Care Planning

Why bother with more effective advance care planning? Studies reveal at despite the person's right to choose end of life care:

- Less than 50 percent of seriously ill or terminally ill patients had advance care directives in their medical record at their doctor's office.
- Only 12 percent of patients with advance care directives had received input from their physician in its development.
- Advance directives were utilized in less than half the cases where advanced directives existed.
- Physicians were only accurate about 65 percent of the time in predictions of overtreatment even when they had received or discussed the plan with their loved ones.

Barriers to discussion with physicians

Medical training focuses on curing. Death equals failure.

Physicians do not want to scare patients or put negative thoughts into their heads.

They don't want to be responsible for having patients give up hope.

They feel these discussions are too time intensive or too idealistic.

The Good News

Only 5 percent of patients found opening the door to crucial conversations to be too difficult. Studies show that discussing advance care planning with their health-care provider had increased patient satisfaction among patients sixty-five years of age and older. Those who spoke with families and physicians about their end-of-life care exhibited less fear and anxiety, felt more empowered over their medical care, believed their physicians had a better understanding of their wishes, and a better comfort level than they had before their discussions.

Starting the Discussion

This may not be the easiest task. It does not have to be formal. It does not and should not be a one-time discussion. You don't have to be old to have this discussion, accidents and disease can happen to young people. How to start?

Questions to Light the Way

1. What does living well mean to you?
2. Are there any circumstances you've heard about on television or the news where you said to yourself, "I would not want to live like that"?
3. Do religious values influence your treatment decisions?
4. Would you want treatments that might prolong your life if you could no longer swallow, if you

were no longer able to think for yourself, or comatose, and not likely to regain consciousness?
5. Who is important to me?
6. What is important to me as my life declines?
7. What do I enjoy most in my daily life?
8. What is the goal that is most important to me as my disease gets worse?
9. For me, life is worth living as long as I can…
10. I want my health-care team and my loved ones to know…

Resource: www.theconversationsproject.org

Advance Directives—you know the thing they question you about when you go to the doctors or hospital. You can get a copy there or go online to print a copy. *Living Will* allows you to have a say in the type of health care treatment you receive should you find yourself unable to act for yourself. A *Living Will* is also commonly known as a *health care directive*. In contrast, a *last will* determines how your estate will be disbursed after you pass. Both documents are a part of a strong estate plan that you make with an attorney. Forms can also be found online.

Medical Power of Attorney (Durable Power of Attorney for Healthcare) allows you to appoint someone to make health care decisions on your behalf should you find yourself unable to act for yourself. This person, as well as your family, need to be aware of the contents of your living will.

Next Step for Making Health Decisions

- Durable power of attorney and Living Will

- The nuances of decision-making: treatment (cure) versus palliation (comfort measures)
- Controlling symptoms: be specific
- Where I want to be to reside

This is not a point in time process, it is an ongoing one. DPOA living will can be amended or modified as circumstances change: death, divorce, disease, important milestones, diagnosis of a serious illness, or crossing the threshold from healthy living to limited health may necessitate a next step plan. Review and revisit with any major change in the last six months or year of life. You need a formal advanced care plan with the physician and is part of the medical record. Some decisions you make may need more explanation so an informed decision can be made.

Code status—CPR (cardiopulmonary resuscitation)

In the 1960s, researchers developed a method of rescuing victims of sudden death known as CPR. It was originally to be used in situations where death was accidental. According to early guidelines, CPR is not indicated in certain situations such as terminal and irreversible illness when death is not unexpected. Myth: people often think it is statistically more successful than it is and are unaware of the potential side effects (too much *Grey's Anatomy* or *Chicago Med*). People are unaware that there are other options for care and deciding against CPR is not the same as not getting treated.

Facts about CPR: patients with the least chance of survival (those with less than a 2 percent survival rate) are those who have one or more medical problems, those who do not live independently, and those who have terminal conditions. Potential burdens of surviving CPR include fractured ribs, punctured lungs, brain damage, never regaining consciousness, risk of remaining days connected to machines, and the reduced possibility of a peaceful death. Options of code status:

1. DNR CC—do not resuscitate comfort care. Comfort measures to meet health needs such as oxygen if you need help to breathe, medicine if you need help with pain or anxiety, and emotional or spiritual support as needed. This is called comfort care.
2. CPR meds—CPR with more aggressive medical intervention and medication to prevent cardiac arrest, but if your heart and lungs stop working, we revert to more complicated measures.
3. Full Code—CPR, breathing tube insertion, attachment to a ventilator, plus medications.

Another thing to think about at end of life is the debate over feeding tubes or no feeding tubes. There has been a number of news stories about this. A better understanding in advance can help when facing the decision. Feeding tubes have been proven helpful to thousands of patients after intestinal surgery, injury, or burns. It is a temporary method of receiving nutrition; however, a patient with a life-threatening or long-term chronic illness often never regains the ability to eat or drink. What is "starving to death"? It is dying due to *forced* removal of *desired* food and fluids. Think of refugees we see on the news. Fact: at end of life, artificial feeding in some cases is more of a burden than a benefit. When a person dies after the withdrawal of food and fluids, the death is from the condition or disease that made the person unable to eat, not the withdrawal of the artificial feeding. Choosing not to force-feed is choosing not to prolong the dying process.

What are the benefits of *not* using artificial hydration in a patient nearing end-of-life?

- Less fluid in the lungs making breathing easier.
- Less pressure around tumors means less pain.
- Less urination means less need to move the patient for bed changing, which can reduce the formation of bedsores.
- Less fluid buildup as forcing fluids in a body shutting down can create an uncomfortable buildup of fluids.

A natural release of pain-relieving chemicals occurs as the body dehydrates. The state that comes with no food intake also suppresses the appetite and causes a sense of well-being. It may be uncomfortable for the family to observe.

The only uncomfortable symptoms of dehydration are a dry mouth and a sense of thirst which can be eliminated with good mouth care and ice chips or sips of water but are not relieved with artificial hydration. Medical evidence is quite clear that dehydration in the end of a terminal illness is a very natural and compassionate way to die (Dunn).

Being prepared with end-of-life decisions can be a relief. For me, having my mother repeatedly saying that she was going to die in December (did not know which December) spurred me to stop thinking about how busy December could be and, instead, showing up at their house in February and accompanying them to the funeral home where we made final plans for their funerals (which didn't happen for many years). I admit, it was a little freaky helping them pick out caskets, choose music, flowers, and obituaries. When we finished, I went home and called my siblings—all who lived out of town. "You will never guess what I just did." Their response was one of thankfulness. "Best gift you could have gotten us." Since then, my brother and I preplanned our own funerals.

Speaking of funerals, have you ever attended a funeral where the officiant did not know the deceased and gave a generic service? If you have a plan for the service, a Spiritual Care Advance Directive, it could include favorite or popular hymns for funeral services, scripture verses, and a list of who is important to be a participant in the service. The "Kick the Bucket" list will be an invaluable tool for the family. Are you aware of "green burials"? This is a natural human thing to care for the person's body after death in a respectful and caring way and then returning them to the earth from which they came. It is ecological and less expensive. No need for embalming the body, vaults, and coffins. No need to keep the grounds pristine—utilizing chemicals and machinery to keep the cemetery looking good. You can find more information online. The more advanced the preparation, the less stress for friends and family when the time comes.

Summary

By having these conversations in becoming informed about advance care planning and advance care directives, you and your loved ones will be assured that your needs and wants are known and that the stress of having to make those decisions when the time comes can be less stressful. It is a powerful way to show love.

CHAPTER 9

Caring for the Person With Dementia

First, let's discuss the difference between delirium and dementia. The terms are sometimes used interchangeably, but they are two separate issues. Delerium is a disturbed state of mind or consciousness, especially an acute, transient condition associated with fever, intoxication, infection, and other physical disorders, characterized by symptoms such as confusion, disorientation, agitation, and hallucinations. The key here is transient – when the underlying problem is fixed, the delirium goes away. Dementia is an irreversible state that progresses over years and causes memory impairment and loss of other intellectual activities severe enough to cause interference with daily life.

TYPES OF DEMENTIA

Alzheimer's – the most common type of dementia accounts for 60 – 80% of cases. Hallmark abnormalities are deposits of protein plaques and twisted tangles of brain tissue. Difficulty remembering names and recent events, difficulty expressing oneself with words, spatial cognitive problems, impaired reasoning and judgement, apathy and depression are often early symptoms. Language disturbances may also be present. Later symptoms include impaired judgement, disorientation, behavior changes, and difficulty speaking, swallowing, and walking.

Vascular dementia (multi-infarct/post stroke) – Second most common type of dementia. Impairment is caused by decreased blood flow to parts of the brain due to small strokes that block arteries. Symptoms overlap with Alzheimer's, although memory may not be as seriously affected.

Lewy Body dementia – Pattern of decline is similar to Alzheimer's, including problems with memory and judgement as well as behavioral changes.

Frontal Lobe dementia – Involves damage to brain cells, especially in the frontal and side regions of the brain due to traumatic brain injury. The frontal lobe controls executive function – judgement, voluntary movements, expressive language, capacity to plan, organize, initiate, self-monitor, and control one's responses. Symptoms include change in personality and behavior, and difficulty with language.

Studies have shown that people with Down Syndrome have a higher incidence of developing dementia.

Facts about True Dementia

Two parts of the brain are dying.

No medications are currently curing it. Ongoing research and funding for research are needed.

It is a chemical and physical change in the brain.

Chronic and progressive.

Always terminal.

DEMENTIA
FORGETFULNESS

Forgetfulness and Memory Loss
Normal

Sometimes misplaces keys, glasses or other items
Momentarily forgets a name
Occasionally searches for a word
Occasionally forgets to run an errand
May forget an event from the past
When driving, may temporarily forget whereto turn, but quickly reorients self
Jokes about memory loss

Mild

Mild cognitive impairment
Frequently misplaces items
Frequently forgets people's names
Has increasing difficulty finding desired words
Begins to forget important events and appointments
May forget recent events or newly learned information
Becomes temporarily lost more often, may have trouble understanding or following a map
Worries about memory loss: family and friends notice lapses

SEVERE MEMORY LOSS

Forgets what an item is used for or puts it in an inappropriate place

May not remember a person

Begins to lose language skills and may withdraw from social interactions

Loses sense of time; may not know what day it is

Has seriously impaired recent memory

Becomes easily distracted or lost in familiar places, sometimes for hours

May have little or no awareness of cognitive powers

90 DIFFERENT TYPES OF DEMENTIA – the most common are:

ALZHEIMER'S - chronic

Early – young onset

Normal onset

Vascular dementia – many mini strokes

Lewy Body Dementia – quicker progression

Frontal Temporal Lobe Dementia – disease of the front of the brain, (Frontal Lobe – executive function).

Other Dementias

SCREENINGS

The screening in the doctor's office is usually rushed. It is not an assessment tool. Only 2 out of 10 people get an effective screening tool.

All real dementia gets worse – progressive. All dementias are terminal. Pseudo dementia – can be caused by acute delirium, mini stroke, or depression. When the underlying cause is cured, the dementia goes away.

Early Assessment Tools

Clock Drawing Test – test for executive function
Mini Cog – if unable to repeat the three words, suggestive of impaired cognition.

Early Intervention

Early Disease management – Provides an explanation for underly signs and symptoms that person may experience. Helps the person and caregivers participate in the development of advance care plans with family, clinicians, and wider support team. Early introduction of strategies and tools to maximize their independence (e.g. daily memory planners, virtual assistant reminders)

Early opportunities to support cognition well-being. Early interventions with nonpharmacological options – such as lifestyle changes, psychological treatment, and cognitive training. May be able to prescribe pharmacological therapies to manage comorbid medical conditions contributing to cognitive decline (think infection, etc.)

Earlier consideration of therapeutic options. Opportunity to consider available therapies appropriate for Alzheimer's. Access to clinical trials with potential to benefit from current and future therapies that address the underlying pathology of the disease and contribute to local research opportunities.

CARING FOR A PERSON WITH DEMENTIA

More than 70% of persons with dementia live at home and family and friends provide nearly 75% of their care. Nearly fifteen million people provide care for a loved one with Alzheimer's or another type of dementia, amounting to seventeen billion hours or more than two hundred two billion dollars in unpaid care. The $202 billion is on top of the one hundred eighty three billion in hospital and long term facility care.

There are ten million women who either have AD or are caring for someone with the disease. Women experience greater incidence of depression, cardiovascular disease, and obesity – factors linked with the development of dementia. Grief is a major dimension of caregiving for a person with dementia, beginning the day of diagnosis and continuing long after the death of the person with dementia. Losses are ongoing in dementia and include the loss of relationships, loss of income, loss of previous lifestyle, loss of independence, and loss of a confidant. Anticipatory grief is used to describe the grief process and has a significant influence on the quality of life for persons with dementia and their caregivers. Often caregivers do not recognize this grief and do not seek help. Grief counseling should be included in caregiver intervention programs.

Toward a Healthy Aging, 8th Edition, Theris H. Touhey and Kathleen Jett.
On line – Teepa Snow.com
Books

Still Alice – Lisa Genova
I'm Still Here – John Zeisel
Where the Light Gets In – Kimberly Williams – Paisley
Surviving Alzheimer's – Practical Tips – Paula Spencer
Slow Dancing with a Stranger: Lost and Found – Meryl Cramer
Gentle Care: Changing the Experience of Alzheimer's – Myra Jones

CHAPTER 10

Safety for Seniors

Influence of Changing Health and Disability on Safety and Security

Physical Vulnerability

As we age, we may become less physically or cognitively able to recognize or cope with real or potential hazards.

Helping an older person to be vigilant about hazardous surroundings, and includes offering suggestions for adequate lighting, placement of furniture and rugs, and markings on sidewalks and steps, and providing information on crime prevention.

Sensory deficits, whether visual (sight), auditory (hearing), or olfactory (smell), reduce the individual's ability to detect dangerous conditions or important threats, for example smelling smoke, hearing the smoke alarms, or seeing an invader.

Tactile (touch) or neurosensory impairment raises the risk of tissue injury from burns, pressure or beginning inflammation that escapes the person's awareness.

External environment Shrubbery, steps in good repair, ramp if needed, porch lights, sidewalk in good repair, motion activated lighting on all sides of the house.

Indoor assessment and interventions:
Home Environment for Seniors

Problem	Interventions
Bathroom	
Getting on and off the toilet	Raised seat, grab bars, side bars
Getting in and out of tub	Bath bench, transfer bench, hand-held shower nozzle, non-slip mat
Slippery/wet floors	Nonskid rugs or mats
Hot water burns	Use bath thermometer, set water temp $120°F$ or less
Doorway too narrow	Remove door and use curtain, get adaptable door hinges, leave wheelchair at door and use walker
Bedroom	
Rolling bed	Remove wheels, Block against wall
Bed too low	Leg extensions, Second mattress, adjustable hospital bed

Lighting	Bedside lamp, night light, flashlight attached to walker or cane
Sliding rugs	Remove, tack down, rubber backed
Slippery floors	Non-skid wax/no wax, rubber-soled footwear, indoor-outdoor carpet
Thick rug edge/doorsill	Metal strip at edge, remove doorsill, tape down edge
Night-time calls	Bedside phone, cell phone, intercom, buzzer, Lifeline

Kitchen

Open flames and burners	Substitute microwave, toaster oven
Access items	Place commonly used items in easy-to-reach areas, adjustable height counters, cupboards, and drawers
Hard to open refrigerator	foot lever
Difficulty seeing	Adequate lighting, utensils with brightly colored handles

Living room

Soft, low chair	Board under cushion, pillow or blanket to raise seat blocks or platform under legs, good armrests to push up with, back and seat cushions
Swivel and rocking chairs	Block motion
Obstructing furniture	Relocate or remove to clear paths
Extension cords	Run along walls, eliminate unnecessary cords, place under sturdy furniture, use power strips with breakers

Telephone

Difficult to reach	Cordless phone, inform friends to let the phone ring 10 times, clear path, answering machine and call back
Difficult to hear ring	Head set, speaker phone
Difficult to dial numbers	Preset numbers, large button and letters and numbers, voice activated

Steps

Cannot handle	Stair glide, lift, ramp (permanent, portable, or removeable)

No handrails   Install at least on one side
Loose rugs   Remove or nail down
           to wooden steps

Difficult to see   Adequate lighting, mark
           edge of steps with bright
           colored tape or paint

Unable to use   Keep second walker
walker on stairs   or wheelchair at top
           or bottom of stairs

Home management
Laundry   Easy to access, sit on
           stool to access clothes in
           dryer, good lighting, fold
           laundry while sitting at
           table, carry laundry in
           bag on stairs, use cart,
           use laundry service

Mail   Easy to access mailbox,
           mail basket on door

Housekeeping   Assess safety and
           manageability, no bend
           dust pan, lightweight
           all surface sweeper,
           provide with resources
           for assistance if needed

Controlling temperature Mount in accessible
           location, large
           print numbers

Safety

Difficulty locking doors	Remote control door lock, door wedge, hook and chain locks
Difficulty opening door and Knowing who is there	Automatic door openers, level door handles, intercom at door
Opening and closing windows	Lever and crank handles, assess need for new windows
Cannot hear alarms	Blinking lights, vibrating surfaces
Lighting	Illumination 1-2 feet from object being viewed, change light bulbs when dim (more than 40 watts), adequate lighting in stairways and hallways, night lights

Leisure

| Cannot hear television | Personal hearing device with amplifier, closed captioning |
| Complicated remote | Simple remote with large buttons, universal remote, voice control-activated remote control, clapper |

Cannot read small print	Magnifying glass, large print books, books on tape/audio books
Book too heavy	Read at table, sit with book resting on pillow
Glare when reading	Place light source at left or right, avoid glossy paper for reading material, black ink instead of blue or pencil
Computer keys too small	Replace keyboard with one with large keys

Fire Safety

Fire-related mortality is three times higher in people over the age of 80.

Risk is greater if medications or illness slows down response time or decision making.

Did you know most fire departments will replace the batteries in your smoke detectors – free of charge. Just call.

Reducing Fire Risks in the Home

- Do not smoke in bed or when sleepy
- When cooking, do not wear loose clothing (e.g. bathrobes, night gown, pajamas)
- Set thermostats for water heater or faucets so that the water does not become too hot
- Install a small hand held fire extinguisher in the kitchen

- Keep access to outside doors unobstructed
- Identify emergency exits in public places
- Wear clothing that is nonflammable or is treated with a permanent retardant finish. Fabrics of animal hair, wool and silk are less flammable
- Use several electrical outlets rather than overloading one outlet

Measures to prevent fires and burns

1. When you smoke, see flames, or hear the sound of fire, evacuate everyone in the house before doing anything else
2. Use normal exits unless blocked by smoke or flames. Never use elevators during the evacuation
3. Stay near the floor because gases and smoke collect near the ceiling
4. In a high-rise apartment, remain in the room with doors and hall vents closed unless smoke is in your apartment. Open or break a window to obtain fresh air.
5. Home fire alarm systems and smoke detectors should have a label indicating UL approval. Smoke detectors should be installed outside each sleeping area, at the top of basement steps, in the bedrooms of smokers, and in all levels of the house. Do not install a smoke detector too near a window, door, or forced air register, where drafts could interfere with detector's operation. Do not install a smoke detector within 6 inches of where walls and ceilings

meet, because air is less likely to circulate smoke to the alarm.

6. Rehearse what to do if clothing catches fire, do not run, lie down, and then roll over and over ("stop, drop and roll") If someone else's clothing is burning, smother the flames with the nearest item, such as a rug, a coat, a blanket or drapes.

Senior Driving Skills and Safety Factors

Directions:

If you answer "yes" to one or more of the following questions, you may want to limit your driving or take steps to improve the problem.

If you answer "yes" to most of the questions, it may be time to consider letting someone else do your driving.

- Does driving make you feel nervous or physically exhausted?
- Do you have difficulty seeing pedestrians, signs and vehicles?
- Do cars frequently seem to appear from nowhere?
- At night, does the glare from oncoming headlights temporarily "blind" you?
- Do you find intersections confusing?
- Are you finding it harder to judge the distance between cars?
- Do you have difficulty coordinating your hand and feet movements?
- Do you have difficulty staying in a lane?

- Are you slower than you used to be in reacting to dangerous situations?
- Do you sometimes get lost in familiar neighborhoods?
- Do other drivers frequently honk at you?
- Have you had any tickets?
- Have you been pulled over by the police?
- Have you had an increased number of traffic violations, accidents, or near-accidents in the past year?
- Do you have any vision problems?
- Do you have hearing problems?
- Do you take any of the following medications: antihistamines, antipsychotics, tricyclic antidepressants, sleeping medications, muscle relaxants?
- Do you have memory impairments?
- Do you have any muscle stiffness or weakness?

Driving

Driving is one of the instrumental activities of daily living. Driving is a highly complex activity that requires a variety of visual, motor, and cognitive skills.

Giving up driving is a major loss for an older person, both in terms of independence and pleasure, as well as feelings of competence and self-worth.

When the discussion starts, be gentle and supportive. Start to test the waters early and gently. There are companies (AAA) that can assess driving ability – impartial/not family. May need to recruit PCP when you go to appointments with your elder. PCP can identify issues related to driving and the older person and the family. It is generally agreed that voluntarily giving up the driver's license is associated with a more positive outcome.

Medication Safety

Age related changes can affect the action of the medication in the body, determines the concentration of the drug which in turn determines how well it works, the concentration at different times of the day, how the drug is taken (orally, injection, IV, dermal, sublingual, etc), where it is broken down, and how the drug gets out of the body.

Comorbidity – Having more than one medical condition at a time. Having multiple specialist for a specific specialty – PCP, Cardiologist, Rheumatologist, Pulmonologist, Orthopod, Endocrinologist.

Polypharmacy – Use of multiple medications for multiple problems or multiple medications for the same problem.

Risks
Duplicate medications
Inappropriate medications
Potentially unsafe doses – remember the reduction in the function of the digestive tract and changes in the other organs that are impact how the medication works. This may mean needing a lower dose or regular monitoring of blood levels of the medication. Gerontologist, a physician trained in the care of the older patient. You may want to explore finding one to use as your primary care physician (PCP).
Potentially preventable interactions

Bring a list of the medications you are taking, including over the counter and herbal/natural medication. Include the dose, route taken, and any questions and/or medical problems since your last visit. If you don't understand what the doctor said, ask him to repeat it until you do. Take a family member or friend with you.

Crime Against Older Adults

May share same concerns about violent crimes as the rest of the population, but feel more vulnerable because of frailness or disability. Living alone, memory impairment, and loneliness may make elders more susceptible to crime.

CHAPTER 11

Spotting Scams and Staying Safe

Anyone ever hear of someone being scammed? Have you ever been scammed? Do you know what "phishing" is? Are you afraid of being scammed? Worry about all the news articles about scams? Let's try to understand this subject and recognize the 3 Red Flags of scams.

"Phishing"- criminals deceive seniors into sharing personal and financial data. A phone call where the caller identifies him/herself as a family member (usually a grandchild) who is in trouble. For example, car break sown, in jail and need money or bail. Then an adult gets on the line and identifies themselves as the "mechanic" or "police officer". Or seeks a letter that looks "official" asking for your information as a first contact.

Scary, isn't it? Older people are targeted more often than any other age group. Here are the 3 basic steps to spot scams" RED FLAGS:

1. If a communication is unexpected
2. Yields an emotional response
3. Urges immediate action

If any or all of the above exits, then it is most likely a scam.

Where to report Fraud

- AARP Fraud Watch Network Helpline – 1-800-908-3360
- Local police
- FTC: report fraud.ftc.gov

Technology changes, but red flags don't

Resources

- aarp.org/fraudwatchnetwork
- facebook.com/aarpfraudwatchnetwork
- AARP Fraud Watch Network VOA/ReSTProgram
- learn.aarp.org/fraud

Tips for Protecting Your Privacy and Money

If you spot Red Flags, disengage immediately

Don't send cash related forms of payment – gift cards, money wired, etc. Gift card scams – scammers get verification numbers from cards on the rack, then put them back. When you go to use them, card is empty.

Don't divulge or confirm sensitive personal or financial information on an unsolicited phone call, text, or email.

Consider putting a freeze on your credit report, which makes it harder for identity thieve to open new accounts in your name.

Equifax: Equifax.com or 1-800-349-9960

Experion: experion.com or 1-888-379-3742

Transunion: transunion.com or 1-888-909-8872

Establish electronic access to your financial accounts which make it harder for identity thieves from doing it.

Use unique passwords and change them frequently.

Scammers – imposter companies or people.

GRANDPARENT SCAM – (look for Red Flags, set up code word – simple and easy to remember, only family knows.) Hang up or use a different phone and call the person who "is in trouble", or call a family member who knows where child is.

Unconventional payment types – gift cards, wire transfers, crypto currency, peer to peer payments (Pay Pal)

Fake social media accounts – very few followers, when was the page created? Has no posts. RED FLAG

COMPUTER SCAMS

"Computer Infected" – do NOT call the number listed. May have a loud, siren type noise. Close page immediately/turn off computer. To remove pop-up, exit browser, restart computer, contact support immediately (Windows, HP, Best Buy). Keep software up to date. Software update is available, either automatically or when you request it. *Any pop up is fake if it comes from a big company – Microsoft, HP, big companies, or the government.

Tech Protection

- Set your computer and mobile devices to automatically update, which can reduce security threats.

- Set privacy settings on your social media accounts so that only people you know can access your posts and pictures.
- Pay attention to web addresses that you visit to make sure you are on the official website. For a business, check spelling, punctuation, refer to other sources of communication (billing statements) or go to the business website and compare.
- Don't click a link or open an attachment unless you are certain the email or text unless you are sure that the message comes from a trusted source.
- Don't click links or call phone numbers on suspicious pop-up ads.

Identity fraud

Done to steal Medicare number, banking numbers, etc. Hang up.

Identity fraud protection: freeze credit reports, create new passwords, establish electronic access on your own devices.

If they say they are from the government, hang up. The government NEVER calls.

Romance Scam

Scammers use deception to create false love interest. Words matter – the impact of victim blaming, i.e. You fell for a scam. How much did you give them? Why didn't you hang up? Place the blame on the criminal. Loneliness can increase susceptibility.

RED FLAGS

1. **COMMUNICATION UNEXPECTED**
2. **CAUSE AN EMOTIONAL RESPONSE**
3. **URGES IMMEDIATE ACTION**

Information from AARP

CHAPTER 12

Senior Living Options/Arrangements

Oh my, its Spring

- Time to get plants, mulch, potting soil, get the flowers/vegetable beds ready

Oh my, its Summer

- Is the lawn mower working; where is the number for the guy who cut my grass last year; who is gonna maintain my pool?

Oh my, its Fall

- Look at all the leaves; the flower beds need to be put to sleep for the winter; where is the number of the guy who raked my leaves last year?

Oh my, its winter

- Where is my snow shovel, is the snow blower working; do we have enough de-icer, is the car winterized?

Is it time to consider living where these projects don't consume your time and thoughts?

- Senior living arrangements options – How do you start?
- Are you looking for yourself, family member, or friend?
- What options are available?
- Do you need immediate services or just starting to look at availability?

Getting Started

- Be clear about your needs
- Are you active, able to drive, shop, dress, and prepare meals?
- Are you starting to need help with medication, activities of daily living?
- Has a situation occurred that medical/physical issues are making it difficult, if not impossible to live safely at home?
- Are home repairs starting to become difficult or just a bother?
- It is time to share your concerns with your family.

Options

- Staying at home with all the memories – holidays, birthdays, new babies?
- Is it a one floor ranch or a multiple story with laundry in the basement?

- It is not how large your home is, but how much space we use.
- It is not how much money you have, but how much you want to spend.

Considerations

- Is the mortgage paid?
- Can you afford to continue to pay the mortgage, taxes, utilities, insurance?
- Are modifications available and affordable?
  - Home elevators, chair lifts, outdoor ramps, kitchen modifications to reach everyday items, widening doors to acomodate wheelchairs and walkers, toilet chairs, handrails, bathroom modifications (walk in tubs, showers, shower chairs, toilet chairs, hand rails, etc.)

Approximate Costs

- Subject to change
- Find prices on-line, at your pharmacy, stores like Med-Mart.
- Examples – electric bed - $2050.00, lift chair - $600 – $3,000 (if doctor writes prescription, may get the cost of the lift mechanism paid for with insurance), wheelchair - $299.00 and up, shower chair - $60.00- $80.00
- What is the resale value of the house when you no longer live there?

Do you have access to affordable services?

- Cleaning
- Transportation
- Bathing
- Meal preparation
- Non-medical help can run $15 -$25 per hour.
- Medical assistance (LPN or RN) can cost $25 - $50 per hour

Time to consider downsizing?

- All of the previous things need to be considered when looking for a new house
- Location is important – close to family and friends, doctors, groceries, senior centers, golf courses, church, and other services

Senior housing option

- Many types available – senior apartments/condos (many with HOA fees and restrictions), senior independent living communities, assisted living communities, and skilled nursing homes.
- Many have vans to transport you to doctor's appointments, shopping, and planned events – ball games, movies, etc.
- Some encompass independent living, assisted living, and skilled care. These are called continuing care communities. These are attractive if your partner is physically less capable.

Benefits

- Living independently, yet having appropriate services as the need arises, can make transitions easier
- Staff will get to know you, levels of care are available as needed, and being close to your partner can be stress-releiving
- In a cold weather state like Ohio, thinking about senior living is more of a need than a want
- Statistically, people who live in retirement communities live longer and stronger

Reasons to live in a retirement community

- #1 – socialization – loneliness kills
- #2 – Peace of mind
- All offer similar services: meals, transportation, housekeeping, activities, doctors, podiatrist, lab work, store, library, and a relationship with a home care agency.
- Meal packages vary
- Meals for visitors is available for a small fee

Senior apartments

- Studio, one bedroom, 2 bedroom is for your personal use.
- The community is yours to use as you desire. There may be patio homes in some communities.
- It is never too late to start looking. Decide where you want to be. Google senior living/neighborhood

- Make arrangements to visit 4-6 places, take pictures, notes
- From there, make your short list – then check them out again – ask for a meal, participate in an activity. These will help you decide if you "fit"

Questions to ask

- Cost plus added fees, Medicare/Medicaid accepted, VA benefits accepted
- Pet friendly
- Walking space
- Parking – assigned, covered, garages
- Family owned (local or out of state)
- Church owned (SEM) may have largeup-front fee, guaranteed residence for life
- Most communities have someone to help with Medicaid application
- Do staff have background checks
- Security, fire alarms, sprinklers, smoke detectors, fire doors

Other considerations

- Transportation – can you drive safely
- Are you financially stable
- Is it time to consider saving for this eventuality
- Include your family in this process

Resources

- Council on Aging – Passport Program, other services
- VA services
- Medicare.gov
- Referral companies – National: A Place for Mom, Caring.com
  - Local: Oasis, Care Patrol, Eldercare connections, homecare services, Local realtors
- Moving and Organizing Mad Easy – Jamie Chile 513-608-4073
- Relocation Planners (auctioneer, realtor, downsizer, mover)
  - Pam Johnson 513-652-0015

References

- Hank Dunn. n.d. "Hard Choices for Loving People." www.hardchoices.com.
- "Conversations of a Lifetime." www.theconversationproject.org.
- Rebecca Pace, CPA/PFS. www.RPaceTax.com.

About the Author

Terri Dixon Gaitskill has lived in Cincinnati, Ohio, her whole life. Married with two daughters, a son-in-law, and three "grands"—Heather, Jack, and Jenna. She loves to read, travel, and garden. Her nursing career spanned fifty plus years in obstetrics, gynecology, and surgery, ending as a nurse educator for the Great Oaks Institute of Technology and Career Development, Mt. St. Joseph University, University of Cincinnati, and Xavier University. This book is a compilation of "talks" she created after she retired to share what she learned throughout her career.

This second edition includes talks I created after the book was originally published. Thanks to friends and others who asked questions about topics they were interested in learning more about that led me to research and present those topics.